Corneal Dystrophies and Degenerations

A Molecular Genetics Approach

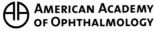
**AMERICAN ACADEMY
OF OPHTHALMOLOGY**
The Eye M.D. Association

**655 Beach Street
P.O. Box 7424
San Francisco, CA 94120-7424**

CLINICAL EDUCATION SECRETARIES

Thomas J. Liesegang, MD
Senior Secretary

Gregory L. Skuta, MD
Secretary for Ophthalmic Knowledge

The American Academy of Ophthalmology is accredited by the Accreditation Council for Continuing Medical Education to provide continuing medical education for physicians.

The American Academy of Ophthalmology designates this educational activity for a maximum of 20 hours in category 1 credit toward the AMA Physician's Recognition Award. Each physician should claim only those hours of credit that he/she has actually spent in the activity.

Each author states that he or she has no significant financial interest or other relationship with the manufacturer of any commercial product discussed in the monograph or with the manufacturer of any competing commercial product, with the exception of Ming X. Wang, MD, PhD, who has been an unpaid consultant to VISX, Inc., and Bausch & Lomb, Inc.

OPHTHALMOLOGY MONOGRAPHS COMMITTEE

H. Sprague Eustis, MD, Chair
Antonio Capone, Jr, MD
William W. Culbertson, MD
James C. Fleming, MD
Carol L. Karp, MD

CLINICAL EDUCATION STAFF

Richard A. Zorab
Vice President

Hal Straus
Director of Publications

Pearl C. Vapnek
Managing Editor

Ruth K. Modric
Production Manager

Design and Production
Christy Butterfield Design

Corneal Dystrophies and Degenerations

A Molecular Genetics Approach

Edited by

Ming X. Wang, MD, PhD
Wang Vision Institute
and
Vanderbilt University

Published by Oxford University Press
in cooperation with the
American Academy of Ophthalmology

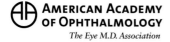 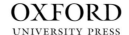

This work is published by the Clinical Education Division
of the Foundation of the American Academy of Ophthalmology,
a 501(c)(3) sub-fund.

Library of Congress Cataloging-in-Publication Data

Corneal dystrophies and degenerations : a molecular genetics approach /
edited by Ming X. Wang.
    p. cm. — (Ophthalmology monographs ; 16)
Includes bibliographical references and index.
    ISBN 0-19-516881-X
  1. Cornea—Diseases—Genetic aspects. 2. Cornea—Diseases—Molecular
aspects. I. Wang, Ming X., 1960– II. Series.

RE336.C6625 2003
617.7′19042—dc21   2002033268

08 07 06 05 04 5 4 3 2 1

Printed in China

To my wife
Suyuan Wang

my parents
Alian Xu and Zhensheng Wang

and my brother
Ming-yu Wang

Contributors

Nancy L. Flattem, MD, MS

Tufts New England Medical Center
Boston, Massachusetts

Beth A. Handwerger, MD

Wills Eye Hospital
Philadelphia, Pennsylvania

Alan D. Irvine, MD, MRCP

Ninewells Hospital and Medical School
University of Dundee, Scotland

Peter R. Laibson, MD

Wills Eye Hospital
Philadelphia, Pennsylvania

W. H. Irwin McLean, PhD, DSc

Ninewells Hospital and Medical School
University of Dundee, Scotland

Francis L. Munier, MD

Hôpital Ophtalmique Jules Gonin
Lausanne, Switzerland

Christopher J. Rapuano, MD

Cornea Service, Wills Eye Hospital
Philadelphia, Pennsylvania

Rajy M. Rouweyha, MD

Hermann Eye Center
University of Texas Health Science Center
Houston, Texas

Uyen L. Tran, MD

Vanderbilt University Medical Center
Nashville, Tennessee

Ming X. Wang, MD, PhD

Wang Vision Institute
and Vanderbilt University
Nashville, Tennessee

Richard W. Yee, MD

Hermann Eye Center
University of Texas Health Science Center
Houston, Texas

Contents

Chapter 3   STROMAL CORNEAL DYSTROPHIES   **45**

Nancy L. Flattem, MD, MS
Ming X. Wang, MD, PhD

Chapter 4   ENDOTHELIAL CORNEAL DYSTROPHIES   **65**

Rajy M. Rouweyha, MD
Richard W. Yee, MD

Chapter 5   **CORNEAL AND CONJUNCTIVAL DEGENERATIONS**   **95**

Beth A. Handwerger, MD
Christopher J. Rapuano, MD
Ming X. Wang, MD, PhD
Peter R. Laibson, MD

Preface

In the closing years of the 20th century, the discovery of the first set of specific gene mutations on human chromosome 5 for stromal corneal dystrophies ushered in a new era for the study of this group of inherited corneal diseases. Using modern molecular biological techniques such as linkage studies and gene cloning, scientists have identified a large and ever-growing number of causative genes. As a result, the study of corneal dystrophies has enjoyed a resurgence of interest among ophthalmologists in recent years.

The challenge faced by today's ophthalmologist is twofold: (1) to keep abreast of the essential new information and (2) to recognize important opportunities for translating these bench research discoveries into new clinical diagnosis and treatment at bedside.

To help meet this demand, a group of cornea specialists and molecular biologists who have been working in the field of corneal dystrophies and degenerations were asked to put together a book on the current understanding and treatment of these diseases. The result of that collaborative effort is this monograph, concise and well illustrated, which captures the excitement and essential new information in this rapidly developing field.

The monograph begins by summarizing the key aspects of the molecular genetics of corneal dystrophies. In succeeding chapters, the various types of corneal dystrophies are described in an anatomically sequential order: from the corneal epithelium, basement membrane, and Bowman's layer; through the corneal stroma; to the corneal endothelium. The emphasis of each chapter is on the current understanding of molecular pathogenesis and its relevance to clinical diagnosis and treatment. Following this anatomic sequence is a chapter devoted to corneal and conjunctival degenerations. Finally, the concluding chapter of the monograph describes the current treatment for corneal diseases using the excimer laser.

The educational objectives of this monograph are to

- Help bridge the gap between the new molecular information and the knowledge base of today's practicing ophthalmologists and ophthalmologists in training

- Assist readers to become familiar with the current understanding of molecular pathogenesis and its relevance to clinical diagnosis and treatment

- Outline the use of the excimer laser for the treatment of corneal diseases, including indications, contraindications, treatment protocol, postoperative care, and management of complications

- Publish an up-to-date guide to the relevant literature on corneal dystrophies and degenerations

With the completion of the sequencing of the human genome in the early years of the 21st century, medicine is entering a new era. Soon, human diseases such as corneal dystrophies may be defined and classified primarily according to the position and nature of the gene mutations and the biology of the altered protein functions.

My sincere appreciation goes to Nancy L. Flattem, MD, who helped coordinate the monograph from its inception; to my mentor, Richard K. Forster, MD, who taught me about corneal dystrophies during my corneal fellowship at Bascom Palmer Eye Institute; and to Francis L. Munier, MD, whose friendship, inspiration, and scientific collaboration I have treasured greatly.

Ming X. Wang, MD, PhD

CHAPTER 1

Molecular Genetics of Corneal Dystrophies

Ming X. Wang, MD, PhD
Nancy L. Flattem, MD, MS
Francis L. Munier, MD

The last several years have witnessed exciting developments in the understanding of the molecular basis of corneal dystrophies. In 1997, the first set of DNA mutations was identified in a gene (*TGFBI**) located on human chromosome 5q for anterior stromal corneal dystrophies.[1] For the first time, the molecular nature of this group of diseases, which traditionally have been known to follow an autosomal dominant inheritance pattern, was revealed. Since that time, ophthalmic researchers and molecular biologists have rapidly built an impressive body of knowledge that has significantly increased our understanding of the molecular nature of corneal dystrophies.[2–71]

Traditionally, corneal dystrophies have been classified according to the anatomic location of disease, the inheritance pattern, and the clinical presentation. However, the characterization and classification of the different types of corneal dystrophies, particularly anterior stromal dystrophies, can sometimes be problematic since they often share common features clinically and histopathologically.

For example, a number of diseases are characterized by Congo red–staining amyloid deposits and include the lattice corneal dystrophies, Avellino corneal dystrophy, and gelatinous drop-like dystrophy. In addition to being stained positive with Congo red, Avellino corneal dystrophy shares with granular corneal dystrophy the ability to stain positively for hyalin using Masson trichrome stain. The colloidal iron and Alcian blue stains of mucopolysaccharides are used to identify a group of corneal dystrophies, but are nonspecific for any one type, including macular corneal dystrophy, fleck (François-Neetens) corneal dystrophy, and central cloudy dystrophy of François.

TGFBI = transforming growth factor beta-induced. In the literature, the gene is variously referred to as keratoepithelin, *TGFBI*, and *BIGH3* (beta-induced gene human cell clone number 3). The latter is spelled *beta IGH3*, *beta ig-h3*, *betaig-h3*, *Big-h3*, or with the Greek letter β for the Roman letter *B* or *b*. The text of this monograph uses *TGFBI*, but the references preserve the spelling shown in MEDLINE.

TABLE 1-1

Inheritance Patterns of Corneal Dystrophies (AD = autosomal dominant. AR = autosomal recessive.)

Epithelial basement membrane	AD	Macular	AR
		Schnyder crystalline	AD
Meesmann epithelial	AD	Central cloudy dystrophy of François	AD
Reis-Bücklers	AD		
Anterior membrane	?AD		
Honeycomb, Thiel-Behnke	?AD	Fleck	AD
		Pre-Descemet	AD
Anterior mosaic	?AD	Congenital hereditary endothelial	AD
Classical form of granular	AD		AR
Superficial form of granular	AD	Posterior amorphous	AD
Lattice type I	AD	Gelatinous drop-like	AR
Lattice type II	AD	Fuchs endothelial	AD
Lattice type III	AR	Posterior polymorphous	AD
Lattice type IIIA	AD		AR
		Keratoconus	AD

Today, researchers are turning more to the rapidly developing field of molecular genetics and are finding that molecular genetic analyses may be not only more useful than the histologic method in defining the disease phenotypes of these corneal dystrophies but also critical in elucidating their molecular nature and pathogenesis.

1-1

INHERITANCE OF CORNEAL DYSTROPHIES

The inheritance pattern for the majority of corneal dystrophies is autosomal dominant, although autosomal recessive and other inheritance patterns do exist. Table 1-1 lists the inheritance patterns of all of the major types of corneal dystrophies. In recent years, linkage and mutational studies have led to the identification of chromosomal locations or genes responsible for a large number of these corneal dystrophies. A significant number of anterior stromal corneal dystrophies have been linked to human chromosome 5q31, and mutations in the *TGFBI* gene located in that region have been identified.[1–35]

Table 1-2 (page 4) lists the 5q31-linked corneal dystrophies based on the position of the DNA mutation in the *TGFBI* gene. These 5q-linked corneal stromal dystrophies include lattice type I, lattice type IIIA, intermediate type I/IIIA and deep lattice, granular, Avellino, Thiel-Behnke, and Reis-Bücklers.[2–34] Non–5q-linked corneal dystrophies have also been extensively studied and have been linked to other chromosomal regions; in many cases, the actual gene mutations have been identified (Table 1-3, page 5).

For example, Meesmann corneal dystrophy has been linked to human chromosome 12q13 and 17q12, and mutations in keratins 3 and 12 have been identified.[36–41] Macular corneal dystrophy has been linked to chromosome 16, and the responsible gene has been identified as the carbohydrate sulfotransferase gene (*CHST6*).[56–61] Mutations in the gelsolin gene (located on chromosome 9) and *M1S1* (located on chromosome 1) have been identified in lattice corneal dystrophy type II and gelatinous drop-like dystrophy, respectively.[44–55,69–72] Congenital hereditary endothelial dystrophy (CHED) and posterior polymorphous dystrophy (PPMD) have been linked to chromosome 20, and there is evidence both supporting and excluding the linkage of Fuchs endothelial dystrophy to the same chromosomal region.[62–67] Another study shows that *COL8A2* may be the responsible gene in a subset of Fuchs and PPMD families.[73]

An autosomal recessive form of CHED (CHED2) is linked to a distinct locus, as compared to the autosomal dominant form of CHED (CHED1) and PPMD, suggesting that different genetic causes are responsible for these disorders.[63] It is interesting to note that individuals with PPMD may have a family history of CHED1, suggesting that CHED1 and PPMD may be genetically related. It is not unlikely that some of these dystrophies are caused by mutations in multiple genes, as is suggested by the linkage of Thiel-Behnke corneal dystrophy to chromosome 10 and Meesmann corneal dystrophy to chromosomes 12 and 17,[1,36,68] although the establishment of the true Thiel-Behnke phenotype in the studies may need further confirmation.

As a prototypical gene for corneal stromal dystrophies, *TGFBI* has been most extensively studied. The gene was first identified in a human carcinoma cell line and later found to be in fact the causative gene for a group of major anterior stromal corneal dystrophies.[1] Mutations associated with stromal corneal dystrophies occur in a minority of the exons (exons 4, 11, and 12) of the gene.

These DNA mutations not only are pointing to a specific molecular pathogenesis of the diseases but also are more definitive than traditional histology in classifying clinical diseases. Perhaps the time has come to classify corneal dystrophies primarily on molecular causation and alteration of protein functions, rather than on clinical ophthalmologic features. In fact, one study demonstrated that the various anterior stromal dystrophic deposits, traditionally considered distinctly different deposit materials characterized by specific histologic stains, are in fact the various three-dimensional epitope forms of the same protein,[74] as expected since these dystrophies arise from various DNA mutations of the same protein.

TABLE 1-2

Anterior Stromal Corneal Dystrophies Based on DNA Mutations in TGFBI *Gene*

TGFBI Mutation	Disease Phenotype	References*
R124C	Lattice type I Gelatino-lattice	1,2,4–7,9–11,13–16,110–113
R124H	Avellino (heterozygous) Granular Severe granular (homozygous) Cornea guttata	1,2,6,10,11,13,15,16,21,23,25,26,29,110,111 35
R124L, ΔT125, ΔE126	Intermediately severe granular	27
R124L	Reis-Bücklers (CDBI) Reis-Bücklers with geographic opacities Superficial form of granular	9,10,28,31,32 15 30
R124S	Classical form of granular	19,26
P501T	Lattice type IIIA	11,13,15,17,18
L518P	Lattice type I/IIIA	3,8,11,12
L518R	Lattice type I/IIIA	114
L527R	Lattice with deep stromal opacities Atypical lattice	3 18
T538R	Lattice type I/IIIA	114
ΔF540	Lattice type I/IIIA	33
N544S	Lattice type I/IIIA	33
A546T	Lattice type IIIA	20
R555Q	Honeycomb dystrophy of Thiel-Behnke (CDBII) Reis-Bücklers (CDBI)	2,6,9–11,15,30,31,34
R555W	Classical form of granular	2,6,9–11,15,16,21,24,26,30
N622H	Lattice type I/IIIA	19,26
N622K(G)	Lattice type IIIA	114
N622K(A)	Lattice type IIIA	114
G623D	Lattice type I/IIIA	16,114
H626R	Lattice type I/IIIA	14,16,19
H626P	Lattice type I/IIIA	114
V627S	Lattice type IIIA	114
629-639insNVP	Lattice type I/IIIA	14
V631D	Lattice—deep	114

References cited only in tables are numbered after references cited in text.

TABLE 1-3

Summary of Non–5q-Linked Corneal Dystrophies and Associated Chromosomal Loci and Gene Mutations (AD = autosomal dominant. AR = autosomal recessive.)

Dystrophy	Chromosomal Locus (Gene If Known)	DNA Mutations	References*
Meesmann	12q13 (keratin 3)	E509K	36
	17q12 (keratin 12)	M129T	37
		Q130P	38
		R135T	36,37
		R135G	39
		R135I	39
		L140R	39
		V143L	36
		I426V	40
		Y429D	39
		R430P	41
Stocker-Holt	17q12 (keratin 12)	R19I	42
Lisch	Xp22.3	?	43
Lattice type II	9q34 (gelsolin)	D187N	44–55
		D187Y	
		D654Y	
Macular (types I, IA, II)	16q22	?	56–60
Type I	Carbohydrate sulpho-transferase gene (*CHST6*)	K174R, D203E, R211W, E274K, Frameshift after 137A	61
Type II		R50C, replacement or deletion of 5′ region	61
Congenital hereditary endothelial	AD: 20p11.2-q11.2	?	62–64
	AR: 20p13	?	
Fuchs endothelial	20	?	65,73
Posterior polymorphous	20p11	?	64,66,67,73
Reis-Bücklers type II (Thiel-Behnke)	10q23-q24	?	68
Gelatinous drop-like (familial subepithelial corneal amyloidosis, lattice type III)	1p31 (*M1S1*)	Q118X, S170X, Q207X, ΔA632	69–72
Cornea verticillata	Xq22 (*GSN*, alpha-galactosidase)	Multiple	87
Cornea farinata and deep filiform	Xp22.32 (*STS*, steroid sulfatase deficiency)	S341L, W372R, W372P, H444R C446Y, IVS8DS GT +1†	115
Central crystalline corneal (Schnyder)	1p34.1-p36	?	116
Keratoconus, AD form	21?	?	117

*References cited only in tables are numbered after references cited in text.

†19-bp insertion at nucleotide 1477 with G-to-T transversion at exon 8/intron 8 splice donor site leading to premature termination of polypeptide of residue 427.

5q-LINKED CORNEAL DYSTROPHIES

1-2-1 *TGFBI* Gene

The 5q-linked corneal dystrophies have been found to have defects in *TGFBI*, which is located in the chromosomal region 5q31.[75] *TGFBI* contains 17 exons spanning 2.7 kb and is induced by transforming growth factor-beta.[76] The 683 amino acid protein (68 kD) encoded by *TGFBI* is highly conserved among species and is expressed ubiquitously in various human tissues, including mesenchymal and epithelial tissues.[75,76] In the eye, *TGFBI* displays a preferential pattern of expression in the corneal epithelium.[76,77] The expression of *TGFBI* is upregulated during development and in wound healing.[78,79] The gene sequence contains four highly homologous 10 amino acid repeats, a secretary leader peptide at the *N*-terminus, and at the *C*-terminus an Arg-Gly-Asp (RGD) motif, which is commonly found in extracellular matrix proteins.[76,80]

TGFBI shares sequence homology to fasciclin I in *Drosophila*, which is involved in neuronal growth guidance, and to OSF-2, a mammalian adhesion molecule involved in bone formation.[76,81,82] There is also evidence that endothelium-derived cells secrete *TGFBI* gene product, and the finding that the protein copurifies with type VI collagen in rabbit cornea suggests that *TGFBI*

may play a role in mediating cell–extracellular matrix interaction.[12,78,83,84] Further work has shown that the protein promotes the adhesion and spread of dermal fibroblasts, but suppresses the cell attachment and growth of Chinese hamster ovary cells in nude mice.[76,85]

1-2-2 Proposed Pathogenesis

An array of DNA mutations have been identified in *TGFBI* in individuals with lattice type I (LCD type I; OMIM[86] 122200), lattice type IIIA (LCD type IIIA; OMIM 204870), granular (CDG1; OMIM 121900), Avellino, Thiel-Behnke (CDB2; OMIM 602082), and Reis-Bücklers (CDB1 or CDRB; OMIM 12190) corneal dystrophies (see Table 1-2). These mutations likely lead to defective protein folding, thus altering the cell–matrix interactions and resulting in a corneal stromal accumulation of mutated gene product into deposits.[74]

It is proposed that the specific location and type of mutation will lead to the differences in deposition observed in the various corneal dystrophies.[74] For example, the *TGFBI* mutations that occur at the arginine residue (R124) in exon 4 eliminate a phosphorylation site, and mutations in arginine residue (R555) in exon 12 affect a coiled-coil domain. These codons and likely other mutated residues are important in the three-dimensional structural folding of the protein, lending credence to the hypothesis that abnormalities of the gene sequence result in protein aggregation and corneal deposition.[74] Immunostaining of corneas from patients with lattice type I, lattice type IIIA, granular, Avellino, or Reis-Bücklers (type I or II [Thiel-Behnke]) corneal dystrophy reveals accumulation of the gene product within the characteristic lesions.[18,74,87,88]

Korvatska et al studied corneas with the R124C, R124H, and R124L genotypes and found that all of the pathologic deposits were composed of aggregated *TGFBI* and that each mutation was associated with characteristic changes of protein turnover in corneal tissue.[89] Specifically, the amyloid deposits in R124C corneas were notable for accumulation of *N*-terminal *TGFBI* fragments, with the amyloid fibrils primarily consisting of a 44-kD fragment. In contrast, the nonamyloid lesions in R124H corneas were composed of a new 66-kD variant, in addition to the full-size 68-kD form. The R124L mutation resulted in accumulation of the full-size 68-kD gene product.

These findings are consistent with an earlier study by Takács et al that identified a degraded 44-kD form of *TGFBI* in LCDI corneas but not present in normal corneas.[90] In addition, immunohistochemistry showed that the abnormal *TGFBI* is localized in the subepithelial regions, including the subepithelial deposits, in dystrophic corneas, but in normal corneas the *TGFBI* gene product is limited to the epithelium. In vitro analysis of R124C and native *TGFBI* peptides revealed the high capacity of the R124C peptide to form amyloid fibrils.[91]

Additional factors are also likely to contribute to the formation of the characteristic deposits. A study by Konishi et al evaluating corneas from 24 unrelated Japanese patients carrying the R124H mutation revealed a continuum of corneal lesions as assessed by Masson trichrome and Congo red staining.[92] The most common lesions identified were large discrete granular deposits in the anterior stroma and star-shaped opacities in the mid-to-deep stroma, but a few of the corneas were notable for diffuse subepithelial opacities in the anterior stroma predominantly, rather than granular or linear opacities. The amyloid deposits in 5 of the 7 patients evaluated appeared primarily in the mid-to-deep stroma.

One puzzling finding requiring further investigation is the report by Akimune et al, who observed cornea guttata in Japanese individuals possessing the R124H mutation.[35] All of these individuals had granular deposits with more advanced disease and a corneal haze. Interestingly, the degree of central cornea guttata seemed to be significantly related to the stage of the corneal disease.

Further strengthening the hypothesized role of defective *TGFBI* in the pathogenesis of corneal dystrophies is the observation of a gene dosage effect. Mashima et al found that homozygous individuals with two copies of the mutated R124H *TGFBI* gene were more severely affected with superficial juvenile granular corneal dystrophy than were individuals in the family who were heterozygous and had one copy of the good gene.[29] Fujiki et al similarly reported severe granular disease with earlier onset in a homozygous R124H individual as compared to the heterozygous parents and grandparent, who displayed mild clinical symptoms.[23] Homozygous R124H individuals have been further shown to have limited recovery of visual acuity after keratoplasty due to recurrence of corneal opacities.[93]

Similarly, in a separate study, homozygous R124H mutations were identified in Avellino patients, but not lattice type I patients, suggesting that one copy of the mutation is sufficient to produce lattice type I, whereas two copies of the mutation are necessary to produce Avellino corneal dystrophy.[2] Based on these data, it could be proposed that lattice type I and Avellino corneal dystrophies represent a continuum of a similar disease process.

If abnormalities of the *TGFBI* gene sequence result in protein aggregation and corneal deposition, it would be expected that multiple mutations in the same gene could lead to a similar phenotype, although perhaps with different degrees of severity. Indeed, this has been observed with lattice type I, which has been found to result from multiple individual mutations (see Table 1-2). It might also be expected that different mutations at the same residue would lead to different phenotypes, depending on how the specific mutation altered protein folding and subsequently aggregation into characteristic lesions. This prediction is also observed in the case of different R124 mutation-producing lattice type I, gelatino-lattice, Avellino, granular, and Reis-Bücklers corneal dystrophies (see Table 1-2).

However, because a single mutation has been observed in multiple phenotypes, as in the identification of the R124H mutation in both Avellino and granular dystrophies, additional confounding factors, such as gene dosage, are likely involved in determining the severity of the phenotype. In light of these findings, the authors of this chapter propose that the *TGFBI*-related corneal dystrophies could all be part of

the same disease spectrum.[94,95] For example, Avellino and granular dystrophies represent different phenotypes in the same disease process.

NON–5q-LINKED CORNEAL DYSTROPHIES

The remainder of the corneal dystrophies have been mapped to different genes and chromosomes other than 5q31 (see Table 1-3). Meesmann corneal dystrophy (OMIM 122100) has been linked to keratin 3 and 12 genes on chromosomes 12 and 17, respectively. Lattice corneal dystrophy type II (LCD type II; OMIM 105120) has been mapped to chromosome 9q34 with mutations identified in the gelsolin gene, while gelatinous drop-like dystrophy (GDLD; OMIM 204870) has been shown to occur in individuals with a mutation in the *M1S1* gene located on chromosome 1p31. The chromosomal region 16q22 has been implicated in macular corneal dystrophy, with a newly identified candidate gene, carbohydrate sulphotransferase gene 6 (*CHST6*), being established.[61] Congenital hereditary endothelial dystrophy (CHED; OMIM 217700 and 121700) has been linked to two independent sites, depending on the mode of inheritance, with autosomal dominant pedigrees showing linkage to region 20p11.2 and autosomal recessive pedigrees showing linkage to 20p13. Finer genetic analysis further identified two independent genes contributing to the CHED phenotype.[62,63,96]

Interestingly, the gene for the autosomal dominant form of CHED appears to reside in a larger area known to contain posterior polymorphous dystrophy (PPMD; OMIM

122000), supporting the hypothesis by some that CHED and PPMD are representatives of a single disorder with clinically distinct expressions.[66,97,98] In addition to individuals with Thiel-Behnke (CDB2 or CDTB; OMIM 602082) displaying the R555Q mutation, a pedigree segregating a Thiel-Behnke–like phenotype has been mapped to 10q23-24,[68] suggesting that multiple genes may contribute to a similar phenotype.

1-3-1 Meesmann Epithelial Dystrophy

Meesmann corneal dystrophy (OMIM 122100) has been linked to mutations in the keratin 3 and keratin 12 genes.[36] Keratins 3 and 12 are specifically expressed in the corneal epithelium and compose the intermediate filament cytoskeleton of the corneal epithelial cells. Mutations in either keratin 3 or keratin 12 will disrupt the extracellular architecture, causing fragility of the corneal epithelium. All of the mutations identified to date occur in highly conserved keratin helix boundary motifs, which are in the same regions found in other keratins to severely compromise cytoskeletal function.[36–41] Knock-out mice lacking the keratin 12 protein possess a fragile corneal epithelium, thus further supporting the connection between keratin 12 mutations and Meesmann corneal dystrophy.[99]

1-3-2 Lattice Corneal Dystrophy Type II

Lattice type II, as compared to the other lattice types, has a different causation, with the impairment of gelsolin, also known as *brevin* or *actin-depolymerizing factor* (OMIM 137350). Gelsolin is a calcium-dependent protein found in leukocytes, platelets, and other cells; it serves to cleave actin fila-

ments to produce cytoplasmic gels. The process is reversed by a calcium-independent mechanism. Gelsolin (encoded by the gelsolin gene on chromosome 9q34) is the predominant intracellular and extracellular actin-severing protein and works on the Gc protein to prevent the toxic effects of actin that occur after being released into the extracellular space during cell necrosis.[100]

Gelsolin has been shown to be homologous with the amyloid deposits found in the systemic amyloidosis of lattice type II (Meretoja type).[101,102] The amyloidgenic nature of D187Y-mutated gelsolin is believed to be due to the introduction of an uncharged polar amino acid (tyrosine) for the acid aspartate, thereby promoting the formation of a beta sheet conformation.[51] In vitro analysis of both of the D187 gelsolin mutations (D187Y and D187N) reveals abnormal processing of the protein, resulting in an aberrant 68-kD gelsolin fragment.[103]

Gelsolin-null mice demonstrate that gelsolin plays an important role in the rapid motile responses of cell types involved in stress responses, which include hemostasis, inflammation, and wound healing.[104] Further, Maury reported not only that patients with homozygous impairment of gelsolin (D187N allele) developed corneal dystrophy of unusually early onset and severity, but also that the corneal disease was associated with severe systemic disease.[105] Proteinuria was present by the second decade of life, and a nephrotic syndrome from amyloid nephropathy developed by the third decade, requiring hemodialysis and possibly renal transplant in the fourth decade.

1-3-3 Gelatinous Drop-like Corneal Dystrophy

Gelatinous drop-like corneal dystrophy (GDLD; OMIM 204870) has been shown to be caused by mutations in the *M1S1* gene located on chromosome 1p.[69] The *M1S1* gene is expressed in the cornea, as well as the kidney, lung, placenta, pancreas, and prostate, and produces a carcinoma-associated antigen. The specific function of the protein is unknown. The identified mutations produce truncated gene products that result in the deletion of a putative PIP2-binding site that potentially regulates binding of *M1S1* to other cytoplasmic molecules or to the plasma membrane. These truncated gene products aggregate in the perinuclear cytoplasmic areas to form amyloid deposits.

1-3-4 Macular Corneal Dystrophy

Macular corneal dystrophy (MCD or CDG2; OMIM 217800) is an autosomal recessive disorder that has been divided into two types, according to antigenic keratan sulfate (AgKS) immunoreactivity.[106] AgKS immunoreactivity is absent in corneal tissue and serum in MCD type I, whereas MCD type II has detectable and often normal serum AgKS levels and corneal accumulations that react with a monoclonal anti–keratan sulfate (KS) antibody. A type IA has been described in families from Saudi Arabia; it is characterized by an absence of both serum and corneal stroma AgKS immunoreactivity but anti–KS antibody–reactive accumulations in the cornea.[58]

Both MCD types I and II have been mapped to chromosome 16q22, and one American pedigree, identified with both types and represented in a single sibship, provides support for the hypothesis that these distinct types are a result of different defects within the same gene.[57,59,60] Keratan sulfate proteoglycans, as the name indicates, are sulfated in the normal cornea, but unsulfated keratan sulfate forms deposits not associated with collagen fibrils of the corneal stroma in MCD type I.[107]

A new carbohydrate sulphotransferase gene (*CHST6*), encoding corneal *N*-acetyl-glucosamine-6-sulphotransferase (C-Glc-NAc6ST), has been identified as being involved in macular corneal distrophy.[61] It lies within the critical region of MCD type I. In addition, GlcNAc6ST activity is reported to be decreased in corneal extracts from MCD-affected corneas but not serum.[108,109] In MCD type I patients, several mutations have been identified within the coding region of *CHST6* that may lead to inactivation of C-GlcNAc6ST. Large deletions or replacements, caused by homologous recombination in the upstream region of *CHST6*, have been identified in MCD type II patients that are associated with a lack of *CHST6* transcripts in corneal epithelium as studied by in situ hybridization.

1-4

CONCLUSION

Molecular genetic techniques are providing an exciting new means for diagnosing corneal dystrophies, as well as offering new insights into the pathogenesis of the diseases and suggesting a new classification system based on gene mutation rather than on clinical phenotype. Mutations in multiple genes or even within the same gene may result in similar phenotypes. Conversely, the same residue in the mutated gene may be substituted by different residues to result in distinctly different clinical phenotypes. Even different numbers of copies of the same mutated gene can result in different severities of a phenotype. While the genetic causes for various corneal dystrophies are still unfolding, it is obvious that these disorders are a complex set of diseases that might be more accurately described in the context of a continuum of a host of DNA/gene mutations, rather than as distinct clinical entities.

REFERENCES

1. Munier FL, Korvatska E, Djemai A, et al: Kerato-epithelin mutations in four 5q31-linked corneal dystrophies. *Nat Genet* 1997;15:247–251.

2. Mashima Y, Imamura Y, Konishi M, et al: Homogeneity of kerato-epithelin codon 124 mutations in Japanese patients with either of two types of corneal stromal dystrophy. *Am J Hum Genet* 1997;61:1448–1450.

3. Fujiki K, Hotta Y, Nakayasu K, et al: A new L527R mutation of the betaIGH3 gene in patients with lattice corneal dystrophy with deep stromal opacities. *Hum Genet* 1998;103:286–289.

4. Gupta SK, Hogde WG, Damji KF, et al: Lattice corneal dystrophy type 1 in a Canadian kindred is associated with the Arg124Cys mutation in the kerato-epithelin gene. *Am J Ophthalmol* 1998;125:547–549.

5. Hotta Y, Fujiki K, Ono K, et al: Arg124Cys mutation of betaig-h3 gene in a Japanese family with lattice corneal dystrophy type I. *Jpn J Ophthalmol* 1998;42:450–455.

6. Korvatska E, Munier FL, Djemai A, et al: Mutation hot spots in 5q31-linked corneal dystrophies. *Am J Hum Genet* 1998;62:320–324.

7. Meins M, Kohlhaas M, Richard G, et al: [Type I lattice corneal dystrophy: clinical and molecular genetic study of a large family.] *Klin Monatsbl Augenheilkd* 1998;212:154–158.

8. Endo S, Nguyen TH, Fujiki K, et al: Leu518Pro mutation of the beta ig-h3 gene causes lattice corneal dystrophy type I. *Am J Ophthalmol* 1999;128:104–106.

9. Fujiki K, Kato T, Hotta Y, et al: Seven different mutations detected in the BIGH3 (kerato-epithelin) gene in Japanese corneal dystrophies. *Invest Ophthalmol Vis Sci* 1999;40(suppl):S332.

10. Mousala M, Dighiero P, Drunat S, et al: The mutational status of keratoepithelin in 26 French families with corneal dystrophies. *Invest Ophthalmol Vis Sci* 1999;40(suppl):S332.

11. Yamamoto S, Maeda N, Watanabe H, et al: The spectrum of Big-H3 gene mutations among patients with corneal dystrophy in Japan. *Invest Ophthalmol Vis Sci* 1999;40(suppl):S563.

12. Hirano K, Yoshihiro H, Keiko F, et al: Corneal amyloidosis caused by Leu518Pro mutation of [beta]ig-h3 gene. *Br J Ophthalmol* 2000;84:583–585.

13. Mashima Y, Yamamoto S, Inoue Y, et al: Association of autosomal dominantly inherited corneal dystrophies with BIGH3 gene mutations in Japan. *Am J Ophthalmol* 2000;130:516–517.

14. Schmitt-Bernard CF, Guittard C, Aurnaud B, et al: BIGH3 exon 14 mutations lead to intermediate type I/IIIA of lattice corneal dystrophies. *Invest Ophthalmol Vis Sci* 2000;41:1302–1308.

15. Yamamoto S, Okada M, Tsujikawa M, et al: The spectrum of beta ig-h3 gene mutations in Japanese patients with corneal dystrophy. *Cornea* 2000;19:S21–S23.

16. Afshari NA, Mullally JE, Afshari MA, et al: Survey of patients with granular, lattice, Avellino, and Reis-Bücklers corneal dystrophies for mutations in the BIGH3 and gelsolin genes. *Arch Ophthalmol* 2001;119:16–22.

17. Yamamoto S, Okada M, Tsujikawa M, et al: A kerato-epithelin (betaig-h3) mutation in lattice corneal dystrophy type IIIA. *Am J Hum Genet* 1998;62:719–722.

18. Kawasaki S, Nishida K, Quantock AJ, et al: Amyloid and Pro501 Thr-mutated (beta)ig-h3 gene product colocalize in lattice corneal dystrophy type IIIA. *Am J Ophthalmol* 1999;127:456–458.

19. Stewart H, Black GC, Donnai D, et al: A mutation within exon 14 of the TGFBI (BIGH3) gene on chromosome 5q31 causes an asymmetric, late-onset form of lattice corneal dystrophy. *Ophthalmology* 1999;106:964–970.

20. Dighiero P, Drunat S, Ellies P, et al: A new mutation (A546T) of the betaig-h3 gene responsible for a French lattice corneal dystrophy type IIIA. *Am J Ophthalmol* 2000;129:248–251.

21. Konishi M, Mashima Y, Yamada M, et al: The classic form of granular corneal dystrophy associated with R555W mutation in the BIGH3 gene is rare in Japanese patients. *Am J Ophthalmol* 1998;126:450–452.

22. Nakamura T, Nishida K, Dota A, et al: Gelatino-lattice corneal dystrophy: clinical features and mutational analysis. *Am J Ophthalmol* 2000;129:665–666.

23. Fujiki K, Hotta Y, Nakayasu K, et al: Homozygotic patient with betaig-h3 gene mutation in granular dystrophy. *Cornea* 1998;17:288–292.

24. Okada M, Yamamoto S, Watanabe H, et al: Granular corneal dystrophy with homozygous mutations in the kerato-epithelin gene. *Am J Ophthalmol* 1998;126:169–176.

25. Okada M, Yamamoto S, Inoue Y, et al: Severe corneal dystrophy phenotype caused by homozygous R124H keratoepithelin mutations. *Invest Ophthalmol Vis Sci* 1998;39:1947–1953.

26. Stewart HS, Ridgway AE, Dixon MJ, et al: Heterogeneity in granular corneal dystrophy: identification of three causative mutations in the TGFBI (BIGH3) gene: lessons for corneal amyloidogenesis. *Hum Mutat* 1999;14:126–132.

27. Dighiero P, Drunat S, D'Hermies F, et al: A novel variant of granular corneal dystrophy caused by association of 2 mutations in the TGFBI gene-R124L and DeltaT125-DeltaE126. *Arch Ophthalmol* 2000;118:814–818.

28. Mashima Y, Nakamura Y, Noda K, et al: A novel mutation at codon 124 (R124L) in the BIGH3 gene is associated with a superficial variant of granular corneal dystrophy. *Arch Ophthalmol* 1999;117:90–93.

29. Mashima Y, Konishi M, Nakamura Y, et al: Severe form of juvenile corneal stromal dystrophy with homozygous R124H mutation in the keratoepithelin gene in five Japanese patients. *Br J Ophthalmol* 1998;82:1280–1284.

30. Dighiero P, Valleix S, D'Hermies F, et al: Clinical, histologic, and ultrastructural features of the corneal dystrophy caused by the R124L mutation of the BIGH3 gene. *Ophthalmology* 2000;107:1353–1357.

31. Okada M, Yamamoto S, Tsujikawa M, et al: Two distinct kerato-epithelin mutations in Reis-Bücklers corneal dystrophy. *Am J Ophthalmol* 1998;126:535–542.

32. Dighiero P, Valleix S, Ellies P, et al: The Arg124Leu mutation of keratoepithelin is responsible for the superficial variant of granular corneal dystrophy. *Invest Ophthalmol Vis Sci* 1999;40(suppl):S332.

33. Rozzo C, Fossarello M, Galleri G, et al: A common beta ig-h3 gene mutation (delta f540) in a large cohort of Sardinian Reis-Bücklers corneal dystrophy patients. *Hum Mutat* 1998;12:215–216.

34. Takahashi K, Murakami A, Okisaka S: [Kerato-epithelin mutation (R 555 Q) in a case of Reis-Bücklers corneal dystrophy.] *Nippon Ganka Gakkai Zasshi* 1999;103:761–764.

35. Akimune C, Watanabe H, Maeda N, et al: Corneal guttata associated with the corneal dystrophy resulting from a betaig-h3 R124H mutation. *Br J Ophthalmol* 2000;84:67–71.

36. Irvine AD, Corden LD, Swensson O, et al: Mutations in cornea-specific keratin K3 or K12 genes cause Meesmann's corneal dystrophy. *Nat Genet* 1997;16:184–187.

37. Corden LD, Swensson O, Swensson B, et al: Molecular genetics of Meesmann's corneal dystrophy: ancestral and novel mutations in keratin 12 (K12) and complete sequence of the human KRT12 gene. *Exp Eye Res* 2000;70:41–49.

38. Corden LD, Swensson O, Swensson B, et al: A novel keratin 12 mutation in a German kindred with Meesmann's corneal dystrophy. *Br J Ophthalmol* 2000;84:527–530.

39. Nishida K, Honma Y, Dota A, et al: Isolation and chromosomal localization of a cornea-specific human keratin 12 gene and detection of four mutations in Meesmann epithelial corneal dystrophy. *Am J Hum Genet* 1997;61:1268–1275.

40. Coleman CM, Hannush S, Covello SP, et al: A novel mutation in the helix termination motif of keratin K12 in a US family with Meesmann corneal dystrophy. *Am J Ophthalmol* 1999;128: 687–691.

41. Yee RW, Sullivan LS, Baylin EB, et al: A novel mutation of the keratin 12 gene responsible for a severe phenotype of Meesmann corneal dystrophy. *Invest Ophthalmol Vis Sci* 2000; 41(suppl):S538.

42. Klintworth GK, Sommer JR, Karolak LA, et al: Identification of a new keratin K12 mutation associated with Stocker-Holt corneal dystrophy that differs from mutations found in Meesmann corneal dystrophy. *Invest Ophthalmol Vis Sci* 1999; 40(suppl):S563.

43. Lisch W, Büttner A, Oeffner F, et al: Lisch corneal dystrophy is genetically distinct from Meesmann corneal dystrophy and maps to xp22.3. *Am J Ophthalmol* 2000;130:461–468.

44. Ghiso J, Haltia M, Prelli F, et al: Gelsolin variant (Asn-187) in familial amyloidosis, Finnish type. *Biochem J* 1990;272:827–830.

45. Levy E, Haltia M, Fernandez-Madrid I, et al: Mutation in gelsolin gene in Finnish hereditary amyloidosis. *J Exp Med* 1990;172:1865–1867.

46. Maury CP, Baumann M: Isolation and characterization of cardiac amyloid in familial amyloid polyneuropathy type IV (Finnish): relation of the amyloid protein to variant gelsolin. *Biochim Biophys Acta* 1990;1096:84–86.

47. Maury CP, Kere J, Tolvanen R, et al: Finnish hereditary amyloidosis is caused by a single nucleotide substitution in the gelsolin gene. *FEBS Lett* 1990;276:75–77.

48. Gorevic PD, Munoz PC, Gorgone G, et al: Amyloidosis due to a mutation of the gelsolin gene in an American family with lattice corneal dystrophy type II. *New Engl J Med* 1991;325: 1780–1785.

49. Hiltunen T, Kiuru S, Hongell V, et al: Finnish type of familial amyloidosis: cosegregation of Asp 187Asn mutation of gelsolin with the disease in three large families. *Am J Hum Genet* 1991;49:522–528.

50. Maury CP: Gelsolin-related amyloidosis: identification of the amyloid protein in Finnish hereditary amyloidosis as a fragment of variant gelsolin. *J Clin Invest* 1991;87:1195–1199.

51. de la Chapelle A, Tolvanen R, Boysen G, et al: Gelsolin-derived familial amyloidosis caused by asparagine or tyrosine substitution for aspartic acid at residue 187. *Nat Genet* 1992;2:157–160.

52. de la Chapelle A, Kere J, Sack GH Jr, et al: Familial amyloidosis, Finnish type: G654—a mutation of the gelsolin gene in Finnish families and an unrelated American family. *Genomics* 1992;13:898–901.

53. Sunada Y, Shimizu T, Nakase H, et al: Inherited amyloid polyneuropathy type IV (gelsolin variant) in a Japanese family. *Ann Neurol* 1993; 33:57–62.

54. Steiner RD, Paunio T, Uemichi T, et al: Asp 187Asn mutation of gelsolin in an American kindred with familial amyloidosis, Finnish type (FAP IV). *Hum Genet* 1995;95:327–330.

55. Stewart HS, Parveen R, Ridgway AE, et al: Late onset lattice corneal dystrophy with systemic familial amyloidosis, amyloidosis V, in an English family. *Br J Ophthalmol* 2000;84:390–394.

56. Jonasson F, Oshima E, Thonar EJ, et al: Macular corneal dystrophy in Iceland: a clinical, genealogic and immunohistochemical study of 28 patients. *Ophthalmology* 1996;103:1111–1117.

57. Vance JM, Jonasson F, Lennon F, et al: Linkage of a gene for macular corneal dystrophy to chromosome 16. *Am J Hum Genet* 1996;58: 757–762.

58. Klintworth GK, Oshima E, al-Rajhi A, et al: Macular corneal dystrophy in Saudi Arabia: a study of 56 cases and recognition of new immunophenotype. *Am J Ophthalmol* 1997;124: 9–18.

59. Liu NP, Baldwin J, Lennon F, et al: Coexistence of macular corneal dystrophy types I and II in a single sibship. *Br J Ophthalmol* 1998;82: 241–244.

60. Liu NP, Dew-Knight S, Jonasson F, et al: Physical and genetic mapping of the macular corneal dystrophy locus on chromosome 16q and exclusion of TAT and LCAT as candidate genes. *Mol Vis* 2000;6:95–100.

61. Akama TO, Nishida K, Nakayama J, et al: Macular corneal dystrophy type I and type II are caused by distinct mutations in a new sulphotransferase gene. *Nat Genet* 2000;26:237–241.

62. Toma NM, Ebenezer ND, Inglehearn CF, et al: Linkage of congenital hereditary endothelial dystrophy to chromosome 20. *Hum Mol Genet* 1995;4:2395–2398.

63. Callaghan M, Hand CK, Kennedy SM, et al: Homozygosity mapping and linkage analysis demonstrate that autosomal recessive congenital hereditary endothelial dystrophy (CHED) and autosomal dominant CHED are genetically distinct. *Br J Ophthalmol* 1999;83:115–119.

64. Hand CK, Harmon DL, Kennedy SM, et al: Localization of the gene for autosomal recessive congenital hereditary endothelial dystrophy (CHED2) to chromosome 20 by homozygosity mapping. *Genomics* 1999;61:1–4.

65. Biswas S, Munier FL, Black GC, et al: Clinical and molecular genetic analysis of Fuchs endothelial dystrophy. *Invest Ophthalmol Vis Sci* 2000;41:S269.

66. Héon E, Mathers WD, Alward WL, et al: Linkage of posterior polymorphous corneal dystrophy to 20q11. *Hum Mol Genet* 1995;4:485–488.

67. Klintworth GK: Advances in the molecular genetics of corneal dystrophies. *Am J Ophthalmol* 1999;128:747–754.

68. Yee RW, Sullivan LS, Lai HT, et al: Linkage mapping of Thiel-Behnke corneal dystrophy (CDB2) to chromosome 10q23-q24. *Genomics* 1997;46:152–154.

69. Tsujikawa M, Kurahashi H, Tanaka T, et al: Identification of the gene responsible for gelatinous drop-like corneal dystrophy. *Nat Genet* 1999;21:420–423.

70. Fujiki K, Ha NT, Lu WN, et al: Unaffected persons with P501T mutation of TGFBI (BIGH3) gene in a Japanese family. *Invest Ophthalmol Vis Sci* 2000;41(suppl):S268.

71. Ha NT, Fujiki K, Hotta Y, et al: Q118X mutation of M1S1 gene caused gelatinous drop-like corneal dystrophy: the P501T of BIGH3 gene found in a family with gelatinous drop-like corneal dystrophy. *Am J Ophthalmol* 2000;130: 119–120.

72. Tsujikawa M, Tsujikawa K, Maeda N, et al: Rapid detection of M1S1 mutations by the protein truncation test. *Invest Ophthalmol Vis Sci* 2000;41:2466–2468.

73. Biswas S, Munier FL, Yardley J, et al: Missense mutations in COL8A2, the gene encoding the alpha2 chain of type VIII collagen, cause two forms of corneal endothelial dystrophy. *Hum Mol Genet* 2001;10:2415–2423.

74. Korvatska E, Munier FL, Chaubert P, et al: On the role of kerato-epithelin in the pathogenesis of 5q31-linked corneal dystrophies. *Invest Ophthalmol Vis Sci* 1999;40:2213–2219.

75. Skonier J, Bennett K, Rothwell V, et al: Beta ig-h3: a transforming growth factor-beta–responsive gene encoding a secreted protein that inhibits cell attachment in vitro and suppresses the growth of CHO cells in nude mice. *DNA Cell Biol* 1994;13:571–584.

76. Skonier J, Neubauer M, Madisen L, et al: cDNA cloning and sequence analysis of beta ig-h3, a novel gene induced in a human adenocarcinoma cell line after treatment with transforming growth factor-beta. *DNA Cell Biol* 1992; 11:511–522.

77. Escribano J, Hernando N, Ghosh S, et al: cDNA from human ocular ciliary epithelium homologous to beta ig-h3 is preferentially expressed as an extracellular protein in the corneal epithelium. *J Cell Physiol* 1994;160:511–521.

78. Rawe IM, Zhan Q, Burrows R, et al: Beta-ig: molecular cloning and in situ hybridization in corneal tissues. *Invest Ophthalmol Vis Sci* 1997; 38:893–900.

79. El-Shabrawi Y, Kublin CL, Cintron C: mRNA levels of alpha1(VI) collagen, alpha1(XII) collagen, and beta ig in rabbit cornea during normal development and healing. *Invest Ophthalmol Vis Sci* 1998;39:36–44.

80. Ruoslahti E: Proteoglycans in cell regulation. *J Biol Chem* 1989;264:13369–13372.

81. Zinn K, McAllister L, Goodman CS: Sequence analysis and neuronal expression of fasciclin I in grasshopper and Drosophila. *Cell* 1988;53:577–587.

82. Takeshita S, Kikuno R, Tezuka K, et al: Osteoblast-specific factor 2: cloning a putative bone adhesion protein with homology with the insect protein fasciclin I. *Biochem J* 1993;294: 271–278.

83. Stallcup WB, Dahlin K, Healy P: Interaction of the NG2 chondroitin sulfate proteoglycan with type VI collagen. *J Cell Biol* 1990;111: 3177–3188.

84. Doane KJ, Yang G, Birk DE: Corneal cell–matrix interactions: type VI collagen promotes adhesion and spreading of corneal fibroblasts. *Exp Cell Res* 1992;200:490–499.

85. LeBaron RG, Bezverkov KI, Zimber MP, et al: Beta IG-H3, a novel secretory protein inducible by transforming growth factor-beta, is present in normal skin and promotes the adhesion and spreading of dermal fibroblasts in vitro. *J Invest Dermatol* 1995;104:844–849.

86. McKusick VA: *Online Mendelian Inheritance in Man* (OMIM). Center for Medical Genetics, Johns Hopkins University, and National Center for Biotechnology Information, National Library of Medicine, 2002. www.ncbi.nlm.nih.gov/omim

87. Klintworth GK, Valnickova Z, Enghild JJ: Accumulation of beta ig-h3 gene product in corneas with granular dystrophy. *Am J Pathol* 1998;152:743–748.

88. Streeten BW, Qi Y, Klintworth GK, et al: Immunolocalization of beta ig-h3 protein in 5q31-linked corneal dystrophies and normal corneas. *Arch Ophthalmol* 1999;117:67–75.

89. Korvatska E, Henry H, Mashima Y, et al: Amyloid and non-amyloid forms of 5q31-linked corneal dystrophy resulting from kerato-epithelin mutations at Arg-124 are associated with abnormal turnover of the protein. *J Biol Chem* 2000;275:11465–11469.

90. Takács L, Boross P, Tözsér J, et al: Transforming growth factor-beta induced protein, beta IG-H3, is present in degraded form and altered localization in lattice corneal dystrophy type I. *Exp Eye Res* 1998;66:739–745.

91. Schmitt-Bernard CF, Chavanieu A, Derancourt J, et al: In vitro creation of amyloid fibrils from native and Arg124Cys mutated betaIGH3 (110-131) peptides, and its relevance for lattice corneal amyloid dystrophy type I. *Biochem Biophys Res Comm* 2000;273:649–653.

92. Konishi M, Yamada M, Nakamura Y, et al: Varied appearance of cornea of patients with corneal dystrophy with R124H mutation in the BIGH3 gene. *Cornea* 1999;18:424–429.

93. Kaji Y, Amano S, Oshika T, et al: Chronic clinical course of two patients with severe corneal dystrophy caused by homozygous R124H mutations in the betaig-h3 gene. *Am J Ophthalmol* 2000;129:663–665.

94. Wang MX, Munier FL, Araki-Saski, et al: TGFBI gene transcript is transforming growth factor-beta–responsive and cell density–dependent in a human corneal epithelial cell line. *Ophthalmic Genet* 2002;23(pp not assigned at press time).

95. Munier FL, Frueh BE, Othenin-Girard P, et al: BIGH3 mutation spectrum in corneal dystrophies. *Invest Ophthalmol Vis Sci* 2002;43:949–954.

96. Kanis AB, al-Rajhi AA, Taylor CM, et al: Exclusion of AR-CHED from the chromosome 20 region containing the PPMD and AD-CHED loci. *Ophthalmic Genet* 1999;20:243–249.

97. Cibis GW, Krachmer JA, Phelps CD, et al: The clinical spectrum of posterior polymorphous dystrophy. *Arch Ophthalmol* 1977;95:1529–1537.

98. Chan CC, Green WR, Barraquer J, et al: Similarities between posterior polymorphous and congenital hereditary endothelial dystrophies: a study of 14 buttons of 11 cases. *Cornea* 1982;1:155–172.

99. Kao WW, Liu CY, Converse RL, et al: Keratin 12–deficient mice have fragile corneal epithelia. *Invest Ophthalmol Vis Sci* 1996;37:2572–2584.

100. Lee WM, Galbraith RM: The extracellular actin-scavenger system and actin toxicity. *New Engl J Med* 1992;326:1335–1341.

101. Haltia M, Ghiso J, Prelli F, et al: Amyloid in familial amyloidosis, Finnish type, is antigenically and structurally related to gelsolin. *Am J Pathol* 1990;136:1223–1228.

102. Maury CP, Alli K, Baumann M: Finnish hereditary amyloidosis: amino acid sequence homology between the amyloid fibril protein and human plasma gelsoline. *FEBS Lett* 1990;260:85–87.

103. Paunio T, Kangas H, Kalkkinen N, et al: Toward understanding the pathogenic mechanisms in gelsolin-related amyloidosis: in vitro expression reveals an abnormal gelsolin fragment. *Hum Mol Genet* 1994;3:2223–2229.

104. Witke W, Sharpe AH, Hartwig JH, et al: Hemostatic, inflammatory, and fibroblast responses are blunted in mice lacking gelsolin. *Cell* 1995;81:41–51.

105. Maury CP: Homozygous familial amyloidosis, Finnish type: demonstration of glomerular gelsolin-derived amyloid and non-amyloid tubular gelsolin. *Clin Nephrol* 1993;40:53–56.

106. Yang CJ, SundarRaj N, Thonar EJ, et al: Immunohistochemical evidence of heterogeneity in macular corneal dystrophy. *Am J Ophthalmol* 1988;106:65–71.

107. Lewis D, Davies Y, Nieduszynski IA, et al: Ultrastructural localization of sulfated and unsulfated keratan sulfate in normal and macular corneal dystrophy type I. *Glycobiology* 2000;10: 305–312.

108. Hasegawa N, Torii T, Nagaoka I, et al: Measurement of activities of human serum sulfotransferases which transfer sulfate to the galactose residues of keratan sulfate and to the nonreducing end N-acetylglucosamine residues of N-acetyllactosamine trisaccharide: comparison between normal controls and patients with macular corneal dystrophy. *J Biochem* 1999;125: 245–252.

109. Hasegawa N, Torii T, Kato T, et al: Decreased GlcNAc 6-O-sulfotransferase activity in the cornea with macular corneal dystrophy. *Invest Ophthalmol Vis Sci* 2000;41:3670–3677.

110. Dota A, Nishida K, Honma Y, et al: Gelatinous drop-like corneal dystrophy is not one of the beta ig-h3–mutated corneal amyloidoses. *Am J Ophthalmol* 1998;126:832–833.

111. Joo CK, Kim HS, Kim-Yoon SJ: Mutations of BIGH3 gene in Korean patients with corneal dystrophy. *Invest Ophthalmol Vis Sci* 2000;41 (suppl):S268.

112. Wang MX, Munier FL, Yang R, et al: Molecular genetic basis of lattice corneal dystrophy. *Invest Ophthalmol Vis Sci* 1998;39(suppl):S1.

113. Nakamura T, Nishida K, Dota A, et al: Gelatino-lattice corneal dystrophy: clinical features and mutational analysis. *Invest Ophthalmol Vis Sci* 2000;41:S539.

114. Munier FL, Frueh BE, Othenin-Girard P, et al: BIGH3 mutation spectrum in corneal dystrophies. *Invest Ophthalmol Vis Sci* 2002;43: 949–954.

115. Alperin ES, Shapiro LJ: Characterization of point mutations in patients with X-linked ichthyosis: effects on the structure and function of the steroid sulfatase protein. *J Biol Chem* 1997; 272:20756–20763.

116. Shearman AM, Hudson TJ, Andresen JM, et al: The gene for Schnyder's crystalline corneal dystrophy maps to human chromosome 1p34.1-p36. *Hum Mol Genet* 1996;5:1667–1672.

117. Rabinowitz YS, Zu L, Yang H, et al: Keratoconus: non-parametric linkage analysis suggests a gene locus near the centromere of chromosome 21. *Invest Ophthalmol Vis Sci* 1999;40(suppl): S564.

CHAPTER 2

Epithelial, Basement Membrane, and Bowman's Layer Dystrophies

Alan D. Irvine, MD, MRCP
Ming X. Wang, MD, PhD
W. H. Irwin McLean, PhD, DSc

The epithelial, basement membrane, and Bowman's layer corneal dystrophies are, at first glance, a confusing group of conditions to classify and understand systematically. In the past 60 years, many authors have delineated corneal dystrophies; some of the dystrophies are apparently unique to the family described, and often they have confusing classifications. In this chapter, the term *dystrophy* is limited to hereditary disorders of the cornea that are not the result of inflammation or trauma. These primary dystrophies usually, but not always, have a bilateral distribution. Well-established distinct single-gene disorders primarily affecting the corneal epithelium, basement membrane, and Bowman's layer include Meesmann, Lisch, Reis-Bücklers, and honeycomb corneal dystrophy of Thiel-Behnke.

In recent years, genetic studies have begun to clarify the molecular basis of several of these disorders, and it is becoming apparent that the classical distinctions between different diseases based on clinical morphology and histopathologic and ultrastructural features are in the main verified by new genetic techniques. For example, the molecular basis of Meesmann epithelial corneal dystrophy (MECD) is now known, and Lisch corneal dystrophy has been mapped to a region of the X chromosome.

The commonly used terms *map-dot-fingerprint dystrophy* (MDFD) and *epithelial basement membrane dystrophy* probably include a wide range of disorders, some of which may be Mendelian traits and others that are not true genetic dystrophies. In many instances, where there is no clear heritable component, MDFD is better classified as a degeneration or a keratopathy. In addition to these primary corneal processes, a number of rare genetic disorders with major features outside the eye, such as Anderson-Fabry disease, have distinctive manifestations in the corneal epithelium.

The group of corneal dystrophies that map to chromosome 5q (including Groenouw type, Reis-Bücklers, lattice type I, and Avellino) are all caused by mutations in the *TGFBI* gene and primarily involve the stroma.[1] Mutations in the *TGFBI* gene have been reported in cases of Bowman's layer corneal dystrophies types I and II (CDBI and CDBII), in which there is some involvement of the anterior corneal epithelium.[2] Reis-Bücklers and honeycomb corneal dystrophy of Thiel-Behnke are discussed in this chapter, while the 5q-linked anterior stromal dystrophies are discussed in Chapters 1 and 3.

In this chapter, where several names exist for the same condition, the *Online Mendelian Inheritance in Man* (OMIM[3]) number and listed name are used to ensure maximum clarity. Other names, which are used less often in clinical practice, are also listed.

2-1

EPITHELIAL BASEMENT MEMBRANE DYSTROPHY

2-1-1 Definition and Clinical Features

The terms *map-dot-fingerprint dystrophy* (MDFD; OMIM 121820) and *epithelial basement membrane dystrophy* have been used as umbrella terms to describe a variety of anterior corneal disorders, including Cogan microcystic epithelial dystrophy, anterior membrane dystrophy, recurrent nontraumatic erosions, and bleb dystrophies. In the original paper by Cogan, white spheres 0.1 to 0.5 mm in diameter were noted bilaterally in the superficial cornea in 5 unrelated female patients.[4] There was no family history in any of the cases. These central corneal opacities were irregularly shaped and did not significantly diminish visual acuity; in fact, 3 of the 5 patients were entirely asymptomatic. Histopathologic analysis showed intraepithelial cysts with pyknotic nuclei and cytoplasmic debris.

Subsequent to this report, Guerry described 9 additional patients with subtle geographic configurations at times in conjunction with putty-gray dots.[5] These map-like figures changed location, size, and shape when sequentially observed over time, but the dystrophy was generally asymptomatic and nonprogressive. The same author had previously noted fingerprint lines in the cornea.[6] Again, family history was not commented on.

Later still, the contemporaneous occurrence of map-dot-fingerprint changes was reported.[7] It is now known that any combination of map-dot-fingerprint changes may be seen at any time, and map-like configurations (plus or minus microcysts) are seen more commonly than fingerprint patterns. Microcysts are rarely seen alone. Maps are characterized as large areas of haziness in the basal epithelium, circumscribed by scalloped borders, often with a clear sharp edge (Figure 2-1); dots are small round, oval, or comma-shaped opacities (Figure 2-2). The fingerprint configuration represents deep epithelial curvilinear and parallel lines (Figure 2-3). The periphery of the cornea is unaffected. These changes are difficult to detect by slit-lamp examination; they are more easily seen on retroillumination or broad tangential illumination.

In some families, the condition appears to segregate as a true autosomal dominant trait (OMIM 121820).[8–10] In such kindreds, the phenotype is characterized by moder-

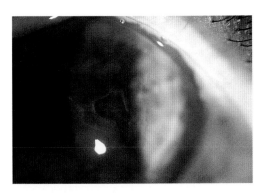

Figure 2-1 *Map-dot-fingerprint dystrophy. Map-like appearance with clearly defined scalloped edges.*
Courtesy Nasrin A. Afshari, MD, Massachusetts Eye and Ear Infirmary, Harvard Medical School, Boston, Massachusetts.

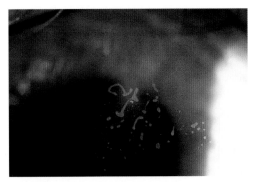

Figure 2-2 *Map-dot-fingerprint dystrophy. These dot lesions appear as round, oval, and comma-shaped opacities.*
Courtesy Angela Ellingsford FRCOphth, Department of Ophthalmology, Ninewells Hospital and Medical School, Dundee, Scotland.

ately large intraepithelial putty-colored microcysts of Cogan or moderately pronounced gray sheets of intraepithelial basement membrane material with map-like borders.[10] Other studies have shown MDFD-like changes to be widely prevalent in the general population, occurring either spontaneously or following insults to the cornea such as trauma, herpes simplex infection, herpes zoster keratitis, recurrent epithelial erosions, or bullous keratopathy. The incidence of MDFD changes has been estimated by some authors to be as high as 76% in the population over 50 years of age.[11] In this context, map-dot-fingerprint changes are obviously not indicative of a dystrophy within the previously delineated definition.

MDFD has been described in patients as young as 5 years, but the more usual age of onset is 20 to 40 years. About 10% of patients develop painful, recurrent epithelial

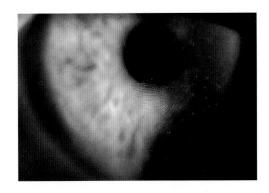

Figure 2-3 *Map-dot-fingerprint dystrophy. Fingerprint lines are clearly seen in this patient after successful anterior stromal puncture.*
Courtesy Nasrin A. Afshari, MD, Massachusetts Eye and Ear Infirmary, Harvard Medical School, Boston, Massachusetts.

erosions, which are the most common symptom. Conversely, at least 30% of patients with recurrent corneal erosions show some signs of MDFD.[12] In a smaller percentage of patients, the mild irregular astigmatism may cause blurring of vision. Recurrent erosions may eventually cease after several years, possibly due to scarring at the level of the basement membrane.

2-1-2 Histopathology

The major histopathologic alteration in the map and fingerprint changes is a thickened epithelial basement membrane that invaginates into the epithelium in the form of multilaminar sheets of fibrogranular material.[7,13–15] Classically, two clinically and histopathologically distinct types of dots are thought to occur[16,17]:

1. Cogan cysts, which are larger and usually seen in close proximity to map changes, are histologically characterized by intraepithelial cystic aggregations of degenerating cells underneath an intraepithelial sheet. They are usually limited to the lower epithelial layers, but may progress through the layers to the epithelial surface, producing clinically evident erosions.

2. A second type of cyst was originally described by Bron and Brown.[13] These cysts cluster closely together and are best seen on retroillumination. In this case, the histopathology is not of degeneration, but rather is of a continuous layer of fibrillogranular material between the epithelial basement membrane and Bowman's layer.[18]

2-1-3 Ultrastructure

Ultrastructurally, cysts can be seen to form within the epithelium below an insinuation of basement membrane.[14] Intraepithelial ectopic extensions of basement membrane and ridges of subepithelial thickened basement membrane are seen. A consistent finding is a bilaminate subepithelial layer of fibrillogranular material of unknown composition.[19]

2-1-4 Molecular Genetics

In contrast to anterior stromal corneal dystrophies, for which the molecular mutations such as those in the *TGFBI* gene have been identified, the molecular mechanisms of MDFD remain unknown. Extensive search for mutations in genes such as *TGFBI* has not been fruitful.[20] The clinical and histopathologic appearance strongly suggests that the molecular pathology in familial cases is highly likely to be located at the junction of epithelium and basement membrane. If, as these authors believe, MDFD is a collection of heterogeneous conditions, molecular analysis should prove helpful in further defining the disorder. Genes encoding protein components of the basement membrane may be relevant in some clinical subsets of MDFD. Large pedigrees in which MDFD segregates in a Mendelian fashion are of great value to geneticists in further elucidating the pathogenesis of this little-understood condition.

MEESMANN EPITHELIAL DYSTROPHY

2-2-1 Definition and Clinical Features

Meesmann epithelial corneal dystrophy (MECD; OMIM 122100), also called *juvenile epithelial dystrophy of Meesmann*, was initially described by Pameijer in 1935 in an 8-year-old Dutch boy.[21] Later, Meesmann studied 3 large German families and reported the clinical phenotype and characteristic histopathologic features.[22] Following these initial reports, MECD has been documented in many other populations. The inheritance pattern of MECD has consistently been autosomal dominant.[22–30] MECD is a bilaterally symmetric disorder of the corneal epithelium, with a characteristic slit-lamp appearance of myriad fine round epithelial cysts of uniform size and shape that become visible by 12 months of age and increase in number throughout life.[22,25,27]

Patients are usually asymptomatic until adolescence, when, in a minority of them, rupture of the corneal microcysts may cause recurrent punctate erosions, excess lacrimation, photophobia, and blepharospasm. Visual acuity may be temporarily diminished during erosive episodes or permanently diminished if corneal scarring ensues. Many patients remain entirely asymptomatic throughout life, with the dystrophy being detected as an incidental finding on a routine examination. The myriad fine round cysts are seen on slit-lamp examination most prominently in the interpalpebral zone (Figure 2-4A) and are enhanced by retroillumination (Figure 2-4B); serpiginous gray lines and small subepithelial opacities

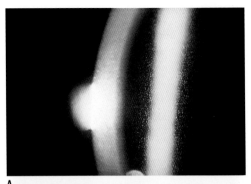

A

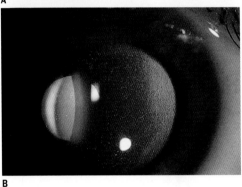

B

Figure 2-4 *Meesmann epithelial dystrophy. Myriad uniformly round cysts are seen (A) with tangential lighting and (B) with retroillumination.*

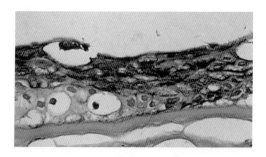

Figure 2-5 *Meesmann epithelial dystrophy. Intraepithelial cysts are clearly seen throughout all layers of epidermis. Rupture of cysts on epithelial surface results in scalloped appearance to epithelium. Cysts are filled with periodic acid–Schiff–positive cellular debris. (Periodic acid–Schiff, original magnification ×100.)*

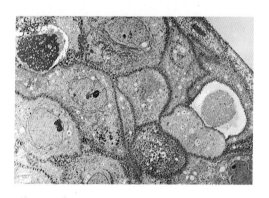

Figure 2-6 *Meesmann epithelial dystrophy. Transmission electron microscopy showing corneal keratinocytes that vary greatly in size, shape, and electron density. Two dyskeratotic cells are seen. There is relatively little acantholysis consistent with largely intact intercellular contacts.*

may be found in advanced stages of the condition.[29] Intrafamilial variation in the severity of disease among affected individuals is well described in MECD and in other keratin diseases.[31]

2-2-2 Histopathology

In MECD, the corneal epithelium is irregular and numerous intraepithelial cysts are seen on light microscopy. The cysts are filled with degenerated cellular debris, which stains positively with periodic acid–Schiff, and the corneal surface has a scalloped appearance due to rupture of the cysts (Figure 2-5).

2-2-3 Ultrastructure

Ultrastructural changes are noted in all layers of the corneal epithelium, but are most prominent in the outer epithelial layers. The cytoplasm of corneal keratinocytes varies in size, shape, and electron density (Figure 2-6). Intraepithelial dyskeratotic cells and cyst formation are clearly seen with cyst rupture onto the corneal epithelial surface (Figure 2-7). Intracytoplasmic vacuoles and abnormally aggregated and clumped keratin filaments that tend to form oval and round intracytoplasmic inclusions, some of which are associated with desmosomes, are key findings (Figure 2-8). Overt acantholysis is not usually seen. The outer layers of the epithelium contain numerous dyskeratotic cells with condensed nuclei, perinuclear vacuoles, and rim-like profiles of condensed cytoplasm. The basement membrane may be thickened (Figure 2-9) with irregular breaches extending into the overlying epithelium, confirming the impression gained from light microscopy.

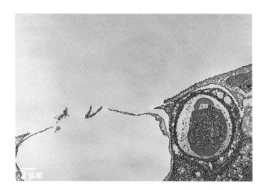

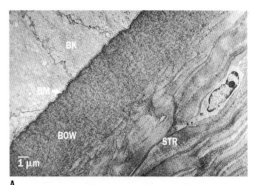

A

Figure 2-7 *Meesmann epithelial dystrophy. In this view, impression that dyskeratotic cells progress to cysts that rupture on corneal surface is vividly demonstrated.*

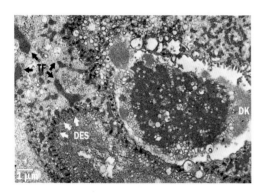

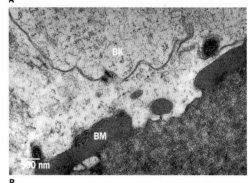

B

Figure 2-9 *Meesmann epithelial dystrophy. Transmission electron microscopy of basement membrane. (A) At lower power, thickening is apparent. (B) Higher-power view confirms basement membrane thickening and shows striking feature of gaps or breaches in basement membrane. BK = basal keratinocyte. BM = basement membrane. BOW = Bowman's layer. STR = stroma.*

Figure 2-8 *Meesmann epithelial dystrophy. Higher-power view of dyskeratotic keratinocyte demonstrating marked perinuclear vacuolization and cytoplasmic condensation. There is abnormal aggregation of tonofilaments, which are seen to associate with desmosomes. TF = tonofilaments. DES = desmosomes. DK = dyskeratotic keratinocyte.*

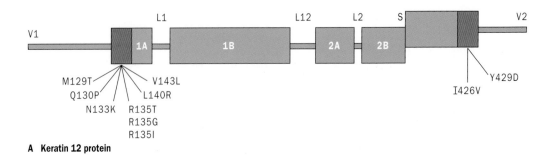

A Keratin 12 protein

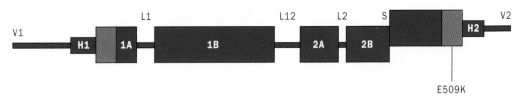

B Keratin 3 protein

Figure 2-10 *Meesmann epithelial dystrophy. Protein structure of (A) type I keratin, K12, and (B) type II keratin, K3, revealing positions of mutations. The alpha-helical rod domain is composed of four subdomains, termed 1A, 1B, 2A, and 2B. These subdomains are separated by nonhelical linker domains, designated L1, L12, and L2. Areas in red at ends of rod domain are regions of high sequence conservation, helix initiation, and termination motifs (collectively, helix boundary motifs), which are critical in filament assembly.*

2-2-4 Molecular Genetics

In 1997, the first mutations in the cornea-specific keratins K12 and K3 in 3 families, including the original family studied by Meesmann, were reported[29] and subsequently confirmed in 4 additional families with MECD.[30] A number of additional mutations in K12 have been reported.[32–35] To date, 11 independent mutations have been reported in the genes encoding K3 and K12 (summarized in Figure 2-10). Mutation R135T in the K12 gene was found in the descendants of the original family studied by Meesmann. Subsequently, this mutation has been found in 4 other families of German ancestry. Using a microsatellite marker within intron 3 of the K12 gene, it has been shown that R135T is an ancestral mutation and that the 5 apparently unrelated families carrying this mutation are in fact distantly related.[34]

2-2-5 Putative Mechanism of Disease

By revisiting the basic molecular mechanisms underlying other keratin diseases, the authors propose a possible explanation for the long-established clinical and ultrastructural appearances of MECD.

While having some unique features, which presumably reflect the highly specialized nature of the corneal epithelium, MECD has many features in common with other well-characterized keratin diseases affecting other epithelia. The multiple cysts seen clinically on slit-lamp examination are analogous to the intraepithelial cytolysis in other keratin disorders, but are seen more easily in the transparent corneal epithelium. The histologic appearance of thickened and disorganized epithelium seen in MECD is characteristic of a keratin disorder.[31]

Cell degeneration is observed histologically in all cutaneous keratin disorders as epidermolysis, typically in epidermolysis bullosa simplex (EBS).[31] Here, in the corneal context, cytolysis is manifested as cyst formation. We believe the periodic acid–Schiff–positive clumps noted by previous authors in MECD represent aggregates of keratin filaments and associated cellular debris. Although keratins are not generally regarded as glycoproteins, it has been shown that keratins K8 and K18 have short O-linked sugar side chains.[36] Glycosylation of K3 and K12 has not been reported. In addition, intermediate filament aggregates have been shown to contain chaperone proteins of the small heat-shock class,[37,38] offering another explanation for the periodic acid–Schiff reactivity observed.

The ultrastructural observation of tonofilament clumping in MECD is again reminiscent of findings in other keratin diseases. In the most comprehensively studied human keratin disease, the Dowling-Meara form of EBS (EBS-DM), ultrastructural tonofilament clumping was first suggested as being indicative of keratin disease as early as 1982,[39] and these clumps were formally identified as being composed of K5/K14 aggregates by immunohistochemistry in 1991.[40] The clumped tonofilaments seen in MECD (see Figure 2-8) are presumably K3/K12 aggregates, although to date the authors have been unable to confirm this by immunoelectron microscopy due to the method of preparation of the archival tissue. Multiple dyskeratotic cells are not seen in other keratin disorders and presumably reflect the unique nature of the corneal epithelium. The appearance of breaches in the basement membrane is also atypical.

In MECD, the authors propose a sequence of events beginning with tonofilament clumping and aggregation, as a result of the mutations within the highly conserved helix termination domains of the keratin molecules. This is well established in EBS-DM, where tonofilament clumps are seen in clinically unaffected areas of skin,[40] in prenatal biopsies of affected fetuses,[41] and in cultured keratinocytes grown from affected patients,[42] suggesting that tonofilament aggregation is a primary process. Subsequently, tonofilament clumping leads to a critical cytoskeletal compromise, with subsequent cell degeneration and aggregation of intracellular organelles. The authors believe this accounts for the appearance of the previously described "peculiar substance" in the cytoplasm of MECD keratinocytes.[23,27,28,43]

The morphologic data presented here seem to indicate that formation of the hallmark intraepithelial cysts is the end stage of a process by which keratinocytes become dyskeratotic, necrotic/apoptotic, and eventually cystic. In a process of increasing nuclear and cytoplasmic condensation, dyskeratosis and apoptosis may lead to the formation of tiny bleb-like intercellular vesicles. The remnants of these dyskeratotic keratinocytes are seen in some of the vesicles in the form of periodic acid–Schiff–positive debris, whereas vesicles near the surface of the cornea appear to discharge their contents. The rupture of vesicles in the outermost layers contributes to the uneven surface of the corneal epithelium in MECD, and this scalloped epithelium may then itself alter shear forces on the underlying cells, potentially exacerbating the effects of the underlying molecular weakness.

A breached basement membrane is an inconsistent finding in MECD and may represent a secondary reaction.[27] Since the basement membrane is presumably secreted mainly by corneal keratinocytes, the breaches observed may be caused by impaired function of degenerating keratinocytes. Cytolysis of keratinocytes, with release of proteolytic enzymes, may contribute to further loss of basement membrane integrity. Breaches in the basement membrane may be the most important determining factor in predicting scarring and, by implication, a more severe phenotype. The reason for loss of basement membrane integrity in MECD and not in other keratin disorders is unclear, but may reflect the unique nature of the corneal epithelium, in which there is centripetal cell migration from an annular basal cell compartment and where differentiated keratinocytes contact a basement membrane.

2-3

STOCKER-HOLT HEREDITARY EPITHELIAL DYSTROPHY

In 1954, Stocker and Holt described 20 affected individuals over 4 generations of a family of Moravian ancestry. Corneal findings were evident in the first few months of life.[44] Clinical findings varied from slight corneal clouding to almost total corneal opacification. Slit-lamp examination showed punctate gray opacities reminiscent of MECD. In more severe cases, the epithelium was highly irregular, with thickened and thinned portions leading to corneal astigmatism and visual loss. Stocker-Holt dystrophy has some shared features with MECD, and its existence as a distinct entity has been a matter of some debate. One study suggests that an unusual mutation in *KRT12* may cause this disorder,[45] although confirmatory data have yet to be published.

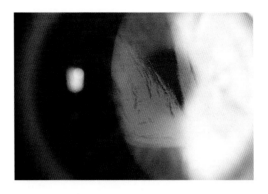

Figure 2-11 *Lisch corneal dystrophy. Slit-lamp examination demonstrating extensive band-like, occasionally confluent gray opacities.*
Courtesy Walter Lisch, MD, Hanau, Germany.

2-4

LISCH CORNEAL DYSTROPHY

2-4-1 Definition and Clinical Features

Lisch corneal dystrophy, a band-shaped and whorled microcystic dystrophy of the corneal epithelium, was first reported in 1992 in 5 family members from Hanau, Germany, and in 3 additional unrelated patients.[46] These patients had a distinctive morphologic appearance (Figure 2-11), with bilateral gray band-shaped and feathery opacities that sometimes appeared in whorled patterns. The cornea between affected areas was clear, in contrast to the more uniform appearance of fine cysts seen in MECD. These changes recurred following superficial keratectomy for opacification. The initial family study, in which there were no incidences of male–male transmission, was followed by further reports of sporadic cases with virtually identical clinical appearance and responses to treatment, including an observed improvement with the use of soft contact lenses.[47,48]

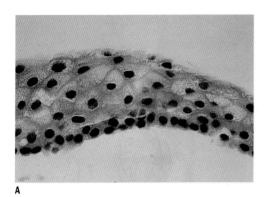

A

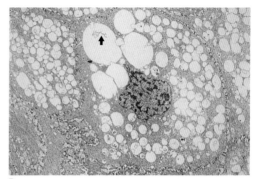

B

Figure 2-12 *Lisch corneal dystrophy. (A) Bubbly intra-cytoplasmic vacuoles in corneal epithelium are clearly seen. (Hematoxylin and eosin, original magnification ×204.) (B) Electron microscopic appearance. In-tracytoplasmic vacuoles are clearly seen, containing weakly osmophilic material (arrow). (Original magnification ×11,520.)*

Courtesy Norman C. Charles, MD, New York University School of Medicine, New York. Reproduced with permission of Elsevier Science from Charles NC, Young JA, Kumar A, et al: Band-shaped and whorled microcystic dystrophy of the corneal epithelium. Ophthalmology *2000;107:1761–1764.*

2-4-2 Histopathology

Charles et al reported the histopathologic features of Lisch corneal dystrophy.[48] Light microscopy showed a transition of normal corneal epithelium into a zone where cytoplasm was distended with innumerable fine vacuoles (Figure 2-12A). Periodic acid–Schiff staining was consistently negative, as was Alcian blue acid–mucopolysaccharide staining.

2-4-3 Ultrastructure

In the same study mentioned above, transmission electron microscopy revealed epithelial cells with tight junctions and multiple membrane-bound intracytoplasmic cysts that were either empty or contained scant clumps of weakly osmophilic electron-dense material (Figure 2-12B).[48]

2-4-4 Molecular Genetics

Lisch corneal dystrophy illustrates the usefulness of molecular techniques in distinguishing clinically similar dystrophies. Lisch corneal dystrophy bears a superficial resemblance to MECD and, before histologic data were obtained, some authors had suggested that Lisch was a clinical variant of MECD.[49] Molecular genetics was used to exclude involvement of the *KRT3* and *KRT12* loci in the disorder and, subsequently, the Lisch locus was identified within or near the pseudoautosomal region of the X chromosome.[50] The Lisch gene itself has yet to be identified; however, the near-completion of the Human Genome Project will undoubtedly accelerate its discovery.

2-5

GRAYSON-WILBRANDT CORNEAL DYSTROPHY

Grayson-Wilbrandt anterior corneal dystrophy may be a variant of Reis-Bücklers corneal dystrophy. The clinical features in the original family were of discrete para-axial and axial gray-white macular opacities. Affected individuals were generally asymptomatic, and corneal erosions were uncommon.[51] As with Stocker-Holt dystrophy and MECD, the issue of whether Grayson-Wilbrandt is a distinct entity or a mild variant of Reis-Bücklers could now be resolved by molecular genetics analysis if the family were available for study.

2-6

REIS-BÜCKLERS AND HONEYCOMB CORNEAL DYSTROPHY OF THIEL-BEHNKE

2-6-1 Definition and Clinical Features

Reis-Bücklers corneal dystrophy was initially described by Reis[52] in 1917 and later by Bücklers in 1949.[53] It is a bilateral and autosomal dominantly inherited disease occurring early in childhood. Patients typically present with a history since childhood of recurrent corneal erosion, photophobia, foreign body sensation, irritation, and pain. Each episode can last days to weeks. The recurrent erosion symptoms gradually subside over the second and third decades of life, with the formation of an anterior stromal haze that compromises vision. Honeycomb dystrophy of Thiel-Behnke was first described by Thiel and Behnke in 1967 as an autosomal dominant superficial corneal dystrophy.[54] Similar to Reis-Bücklers, this dystrophy also begins in childhood with a progressive history of recurrent corneal erosion into young adulthood that subsides with the formation of anterior stromal scarring later in life.

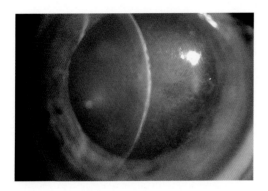

Figure 2-13 *Reis-Bücklers corneal dystrophy. Reticular pattern and anterior opacity and irregularity can be seen in this slit-lamp photograph.*
Courtesy Richard K. Forster, MD, Bascom Palmer Eye Institute, Miami, Florida.

Clinically, Reis-Bücklers corneal dystrophy is characterized by a fine reticular pattern of opacities in Bowman's layer (Figure 2-13). After numerous episodes of recurrent corneal erosion, the anterior cornea gradually becomes scarred and superficial gray-white opacities become mixed with the original reticular pattern. Over time, the corneal surface becomes more irregular and opacified, decreasing vision. Honeycomb dystrophy of Thiel-Behnke presents with similar clinical features, with a notable feature of honeycomb-like gray-white opacities in Bowman's layer (Figure 2-14). Recurrent erosion and progressive scarring result in clouding and opacification of the anterior corneal stroma, which in turn result in reduced vision, as in Reis-Bücklers.

2-6-2 Histopathology

Histopathologically, Reis-Bücklers dystrophy is characterized by pea-like projections from Bowman's layer extending into the epithelium. Often, Bowman's layer is absent in many areas, presumably because of recurrent destruction and injury secondary to erosion and replacement by fibrocellular connective tissue.[55] In honeycomb dystrophy of Thiel-Behnke, similar nodular projections into the epithelium were noted with the thickened and duplicated epithelial basement membrane.[56]

2-6-3 Ultrastructure

At the ultrastructural level, the fibrocellular material that replaces Bowman's layer consists of collagen fibrils ranging in diameter from 80 to 400 Å. The fibrocellular material accumulates between Bowman's layer and corneal epithelium where Bowman's layer is intact.[57] The primary pathophysiologic event that gives rise to these two diseases has not been identified. It has been proposed that the primary defect is either in superficial keratocytes, producing abnormal collagen fibrils that damage Bowman's layer, or in epithelial cells with recurrent erosion leading to deposition of fibrocellular material and destruction of Bowman's layer.[58,59]

2-6-4 Molecular Genetics

The identification of the first set of causative gene mutation for anterior stromal corneal dystrophies[1] significantly advanced our understanding of the molecular cause of these diseases. It now appears that there are at least two distinct DNA mutations in the *TGFBI* gene on human chromosome 5 that may be causative for both Reis-Bücklers and honeycomb dystrophy of Thiel-Behnke: R555Q and R124L (see Table 1-2 in Chapter 1). The superficial variant of granular dystrophy also appears to share the R124L mutation. In addition to the 5q31 locus, a pedigree segregating a Thiel-Behnke–like phenotype has been mapped to the 10q23-24 region,[60] suggesting that the disease may be caused by multiple genes.

It has been proposed that in cases where the *TGFBI* gene is implicated, the DNA point mutations result in the synthesis of an abnormal form of this protein by the epithelial cells, leading to misfolding of the protein and deposition in the cornea.[61] Epithelial and basement membrane abnormality leads to recurrent erosion and reactive fibrocellular infiltration and absorption of Bowman's layer. Further molecular biological study of these dystrophies will help differentiate and possibly reclassify these dystrophies based on molecular defect.

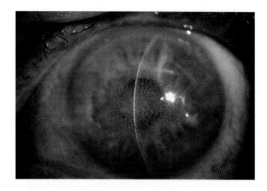

Figure 2-14 *Honeycomb dystrophy of Thiel-Behnke. Characteristic honeycomb pattern can be seen in anterior corneal stroma, with irregularly raised anterior surface due to recurrent erosion and scarring. Courtesy Richard K. Forster, MD, Bascom Palmer Eye Institute, Miami, Florida.*

CORNEAL EPITHELIAL DYSTROPHIES ASSOCIATED WITH GENETIC DISEASE

The cornea shares an ectodermal origin with the skin, and one consequence of this common ontogeny is that a number of genodermatoses have corneal manifestations, which, in some cases, are virtually diagnostic of the underlying disease. Many other systemic diseases have characteristic corneal epithelial appearances. These conditions are not primarily corneal processes and are therefore not strictly corneal dystrophies but, in order to provide a comprehensive account of inherited corneal disorders, brief descriptions are included here.

2-7-1 Anderson-Fabry Disease

Fabry disease (OMIM 301500), or cornea verticillata, is an X-linked lysosomal storage disease resulting from absence of a specific alpha-galactosidase, lysosomal ceramide trihexosidase. Mutations in the alpha-galactosidase A gene (*GLA*) underscore the biochemical abnormalities.[62] The excess neutral glycosphingolipids are deposited in many tissues, including the blood vessels, neurologic tissue, kidneys, and cornea. In male hemizygotes, death is usually secondary to renal failure or to cardiac or cerebrovascular disease.

The most striking clinical feature is diffuse angiokeratomas of the skin that can be very extensive, and the initial presentation is often with a characteristic burning pain in the extremities (acroparesthesia). Affected male hemizygotes and, to a lesser extent, female carriers develop a characteristic appearance of fine whorled subepithelial lines radiating from a common point in the cornea (the name *verticillata* or *vortex dystrophy* vividly evokes the clinical appearance). These changes may appear as early as age 6 months[63] and, in some cases, are sufficient to make the diagnosis.[64] Electron microscopy of the corneal epithelium reveals multiple intracytoplasmic bodies, which are also seen within the stromal keratocytes. The ultrastructural appearance of subepithelial ridges or duplications of the basement membrane may explain the whorled lines.

2-7-2 Keratosis Follicularis Spinulosa Decalvans

Keratosis follicularis spinulosa decalvans (KFSD; OMIM 308800) is an X-linked recessive disorder of epithelial tissue initially described in 1926 by the eminent Dutch dermatologist Siemens.[65] All cases reported since then have been in patients of Dutch origin. The most striking clinical appearance of these patients is loss of hair, especially of the scalp, eyebrows, and eyelashes. Patients are often atopic and complain of photophobia.

The corneal appearance is of punctate farinaceous opacities within and beneath the epithelium (Figure 2-15). Female heterozygotes may exhibit minor forms of these corneal anomalies. The corneal histopathology and ultrastructure of KFSD have not been well studied, but the few reports that exist describe large vacuolated cells within the superficial corneal epithelium, with eosinophilic contents and pyknotic nuclei. Epithelial basement membrane thickening has also been noted. The KFSD gene has been mapped to Xp22.13-p22.2 in several Dutch kindreds.[66] It is interesting to note that the KFSD gene is mapped to the same locus as Lisch corneal dystrophy, suggesting that these two distinctly different clinical entities may be caused by molecular defects in the same gene.

2-7-3 Epidermolysis Bullosa

Epidermolysis bullosa (EB) encompasses a number of clinical and genetically distinct subtypes of epidermal fragility disorders, classified by the level of fragility. The most superficial, EB simplex, is characterized by intraepithelial cell lysis; junctional EB is characterized by lysis through the dermo–epidermal junction (DEJ); and in dystrophic EB, the defect is below the DEJ. The molecular pathology of this group of conditions is well established,[67] and many of the molecules involved are expressed in the cornea.

Corneal involvement has been reported in all EB subtypes,[68] and corneal epithelial dystrophy has been described in severe forms of EB simplex, caused by mutations in the basal keratin genes *KRT5* and *KRT14*. Even in severe cases of EB simplex, corneal findings are not prominent, but do sometimes occur as a ring-like configuration of fine bullous lesions in the midperiphery bilaterally at the level of deep corneal epithelium superficial to Bowman's layer.[69] This is consistent with the known corneal expression pattern of K5 and K14, which are expressed in keratinocytes of the limbus, but not in the central cornea, where K3 and K12 are the predominant keratin pair.

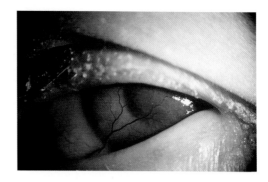

Figure 2-15 *Keratosis follicularis spinulosa decalvans. Extensive punctate farinaceous intraepithelial opacities.*

Courtesy Gabriele Richard, MD, Thomas Jefferson University, Philadelphia, Pennsylvania.

2-7-4 Corneodermato-osseous Syndrome

Corneodermato-osseous syndrome (OMIM 122440) has been described in a single family. The kindred included 7 affected persons in 3 generations, and there were 3 instances of male–male transmission. The affected phenotype included diffuse palmoplantar hyperkeratosis, distal onycholysis, brachydactyly, short stature, and dental problems.[70] Most patients complained of photophobia and watering of the eyes and, in 1 patient, the condition was sufficiently severe to warrant a corneal graft, although the changes recurred in the graft.

2-7-5 Darier Disease

Darier disease (OMIM 124200) is an autosomal dominant genodermatosis characterized by pigmented warty papules prominent over the intertriginous areas, scalp, and forehead. Palmar and plantar pits are common manifestations, as is nail dystrophy. Corneal epithelial manifestations are not commonly a clinical problem, but a characteristic pattern of involvement is recognized, consisting of flat nebular intraepithelial opacities in the peripheral cornea, separated from the limbus by a lucid zone. These changes are best seen with broad oblique examination. Histopathology of biopsied material has shown epithelial basal cell edema, with deposition of a granular material beneath the basement membrane.

A lack of hemidesmosomes and a multilaminate basement membrane were also noted.[71]

Darier disease is caused by mutations in *ATP2A2*, which encodes for a sarco/endoplasmic reticulum calcium pump thought to be important in desmosome assembly.[72] Intracellular calcium is an important factor in epithelial differentiation, and so the corneal defects seen, like those of the epidermis, are presumably secondary to the primary genetic defect affecting calcium metabolism.

2-7-6 Hereditary Mucoepithelial Dysplasia

Hereditary mucoepithelial dysplasia (OMIM 158310) is a rare autosomal dominant disorder with dermatologic, ocular, and pulmonary manifestations, the latter being the most common cause of death.[73,74] Ocular changes begin in childhood, and the corneal epithelium contains multiple microcysts, which may accumulate at the limbus. Corneal pannus formation and advanced subcapsular cataracts lead to legal blindness within the first decade of life. Histopathology demonstrates varied thickness of the corneal epithelium, intraepithelial dyskeratotic bodies, and lack of normal desmosomes and gap junctions.[74]

2-7-7 Richner-Hanhart Syndrome

Richner-Hanhart syndrome (OMIM 276600), also known as *tyrosine transaminase deficiency* or *keratosis palmaris et plantaris with corneal dystrophy*, is a rare autosomal recessive disorder characterized by corneal lesions, palmar and plantar keratoses, and mental retardation. Herpetiform central epithelial opacities appear early in the course of the disease[75] and may be associated with recurrent episodes of photophobia and increased lacrimation. In some cases, the skin alterations occur in the absence of corneal lesions.[76] Histopathology shows hyperplastic stratified epithelium with intracellular edema.[77]

2-8

GENERAL PRINCIPLES OF MANAGEMENT

2-8-1 Supportive Treatment

The primary corneal epithelial dystrophies are systemic genetic conditions in which the limbal stem cells harbor the underlying mutation. As a consequence, the reports of unsuccessful corneal grafting in Meesmann dystrophy and other dystrophies are not surprising. Therefore, current management is aimed at the amelioration of symptoms and maintenance of vision, rather than at a definitive curative surgical procedure.

The mild astigmatism and associated blurring of vision in map-dot-fingerprint dystrophy (MDFD) may be treated with topical hypertonic saline (cream or drops), which may decrease epithelial edema and irregularity. If the astigmatism is more marked, the central epithelium can be removed carefully with a moist cotton applicator. For symptomatic recurrent corneal erosions, a loose-fitting high water-content soft contact lens is helpful in reducing recurrence. Placement of the lens may cause initial corneal inflammation and edema, which can be ameliorated with cycloplegics and low-dose corticosteroids. This reaction usually resolves within a few days. The lens should be left in place for up to 3 months to enable stable reattachment of the basal layer to the basement membrane. Oral tetracycline antibiotics may also be used with varying degrees of success in recalcitrant cases.

2-8-2 Anterior Stromal Puncture and Phototherapeutic Keratoplasty

Anterior stromal needle puncture is an established treatment for recurrent corneal erosions, although the treatment has limited efficacy and is not applicable to lesions in the visual axis. In recent years, phototherapeutic keratoplasty has been increasingly used both for recalcitrant recurrent corneal erosions and for the more severe forms of epithelial corneal dystrophy. In the true genetic dystrophies, the condition always recurs to some extent, although it may be less severe after treatment.

2-8-3 Possibilities for Gene Therapy

The cornea has a relatively small, easily accessible total area, making it attractive for gene therapy. The well-defined location of the stem cells within the limbal region should also make the cornea a good candidate tissue, as it should be possible to target these cells through in vivo approaches.[78] Currently, the major obstacle to successful gene therapy for epidermal diseases is the issue of stem cell targeting. Stem cells must be treated since more differentiated cells would lose any transgene at the time of cell death. A further technical difficulty is the introduction of the foreign DNA/gene into the target cells. These approaches usually involve viral vectors such as retroviruses, adenoviruses, and adeno-associated viruses. These possible modalities have the theoretical difficulties of inducing an immune response to the virally infected cell and the outside possibility of generating replication-competent viruses, which could lead to insertional mutations in the host genome.

Because of these major problems, gene therapy is unlikely to become a therapeutic option for diseases involving widespread structural molecules that are expressed at high levels and that have dominant-negative pathologies, such as Meesmann epithelial corneal dystrophy (MECD). In theory, recessive diseases may be better targets for gene therapy approaches, but these are rare in the cornea.

To develop gene therapy for corneal epithelial dystrophies, it is essential that realistic animal models be available. A mouse model resembling MECD has been made by targeted ablation of the murine K12 gene.[79] Although these mice have a very fragile corneal epithelium due to complete absence of the K3/K12 cytoskeleton, they are not a good model for dominant-acting mutations in the K3 or K12 genes, as seen in MECD. Further animal models of corneal dystrophies will have to be made by "knock-in" gene targeting methods or conventional transgenics.

A more fundamental problem exists in the development of gene therapy for corneal disorders. In dominant disorders such as MECD, powerful dominant-negative interference is exerted by the mutant polypeptide. Consequently, conventional gene replacement therapy methods, which are suitable for recessive diseases, are not appropriate. One method under development in the authors' group for keratin disorders, including MECD, is the use of specific ribozymes, based on the system described by Montgomery and Dietz for the fibrillin gene.[80] These small RNA molecules can be designed specifically to cleave mRNA species at user-defined sequences. Thus, ribozymes can be used to target specific mutant mRNAs, common polymorphisms linked to mutations, or to eliminate all endogenous mRNA and simultaneously replace it with a modified mRNA.[81] It remains to be seen whether this technology develops into clinically useful applications.

2-9

CONCLUSION

Tremendous advances have been made in recent years in unraveling the molecular basis of genetic diseases of the corneal epithelium, basement membrane, and Bowman's layer. Understanding the molecular genetics will undoubtedly help in the correct diagnosis and genetic counseling of patients and their families. However, there is much still to be done. The more heterogeneous disorders such as MDFD have yet to be tackled, and positional cloning of linked genes, such as that for Lisch dystrophy, has yet to be completed. The rapid progress made in decoding the human genome is certain to lead to the identification of all or most corneal disease genes in the coming decade.

Gene therapy development is at a very early stage. True animal models carrying murine equivalents of human mutations must be generated, and numerous technical problems in the design and delivery of therapeutic genes have yet to be solved. Since corneal dystrophies are not life-threatening, prenatal diagnosis leading to termination of pregnancy is unlikely ever to gain approval. Preimplantation diagnosis is one way around this ethical problem; however, the technology is technically demanding, very expensive, and proving difficult to put into common practice. Therefore, the development of gene therapy offers the only hope of permanently treating inherited disorders of the corneal epithelium, basement membrane, and Bowman's layer. This, together with the fact that the cornea is a small accessible tissue, means that corneal gene therapy is likely to receive a great deal of attention over the next few years.

ACKNOWLEDGMENT

Dr Irvine and Professor McLean wish to thank the patients and their families who took part in their corneal research projects. The original studies in the Epithelial Genetics Group laboratories were funded by the Wellcome Trust and the Dystrophic Epidermolysis Bullosa Research Association. Professor McLean is currently supported by a Wellcome Trust Senior Research Fellowship.

REFERENCES

1. Munier FL, Korvatska E, Djemai A, et al: Kerato-epithelin mutations in four 5q31-linked corneal dystrophies. *Nat Genet* 1997;15:247–251.

2. Ridgway AE, Akhtar S, Munier FL, et al: Ultrastructural and molecular analysis of Bowman's layer corneal dystrophies: an epithelial origin? *Invest Ophthalmol Vis Sci* 2000;41:3286–3292.

3. McKusick VA: *Online Mendelian Inheritance in Man* (OMIM). Center for Medical Genetics, Johns Hopkins University, and National Center for Biotechnology Information, National Library of Medicine, 2002. www.ncbi.nlm.nih.gov/omim

4. Cogan DG: Microcystic dystrophy of the corneal epithelium. *Trans Am Ophthalmol Soc* 1964;62:213–216.

5. Guerry D III: Observations on Cogan's microcystic dystrophy of the corneal epithelium. *Trans Am Ophthalmol Soc* 1965;63:320–334.

6. Guerry D III: Fingerprint lines in the cornea. *Am J Ophthalmol* 1950;33:724–727.

7. Laibson PR: Microcystic corneal dystrophy. *Trans Am Ophthalmol Soc* 1976;74:488–531.

8. Franceschetti A: [Hereditary recurrent erosion of the cornea.] *Z Augenheilkd* 1928;66: 309–313.

9. Bron AJ, Burgess SE: Inherited recurrent corneal erosion. *Trans Ophthalmol Soc U K* 1981;101: 239–243.

10. Laibson PR, Krachmer JH: Familial occurrence of dot (microcystic), map, fingerprint dystrophy of the cornea. *Invest Ophthalmol* 1975;14: 397–399.

11. Werblin TP, Hirst LW, Stark WJ, et al: Prevalence of map-dot-fingerprint changes in the cornea. *Br J Ophthalmol* 1981;65:401–409.

12. Reidy JJ, Paulus MP, Gona S: Recurrent erosions of the cornea: epidemiology and treatment. *Cornea* 2000;19:767–771.

13. Bron AJ, Brown NA: Some superficial corneal disorders. *Trans Ophthalmol Soc U K* 1971; 91:XII+.

14. Cogan DG, Kuwabara T, Donaldson DD, et al: Microcystic dystrophy of the cornea: a partial explanation for its pathogenesis. *Arch Ophthalmol* 1974;92:470–474.

15. Rodrigues MM, Fine BS, Laibson PR, et al: Disorders of the corneal epithelium: a clinico-pathologic study of dot, geographic, and fingerprint patterns. *Arch Ophthalmol* 1974;92:475–482.

16. Bron AJ, Tripathi RC: Cystic disorders of the corneal epithelium, I: clinical aspects. *Br J Ophthalmol* 1973;57:361–375.

17. Tripathi RC, Bron AJ: Cystic disorders of the corneal epithelium, II: pathogenesis. *Br J Ophthalmol* 1973;57:376–390.

18. Dark AJ: Bleb dystrophy of the cornea: histochemistry and ultrastructure. *Br J Ophthalmol* 1977;61:65–69.

19. Dark AJ: Cogan's microcystic dystrophy of the cornea: ultrastructure and photomicroscopy. *Br J Ophthalmol* 1978;62:821–830.

20. Wang MX, Munier FL, Yang R, et al: BIGH3 mutations are not present in patients with map-dot-fingerprint corneal dystrophy. Presented at Ophthalmic Genetics Club, American Academy of Ophthalmology Annual Meeting, New Orleans, 1998.

21. Pameijer JK: [About a strange familial surface change of the cornea.] *Klin Monatsbl Augenheilkd* 1935;103:516–517.

22. Meesmann A, Wilke F: [Clinical and anatomic studies about a hitherto unknown dominantly inherited epithelial dystrophy of the cornea.] *Klin Monatsbl Augenheilkd* 1939;103: 361–391.

23. Kuwabara T, Ciccarelli EC: Meesmann's corneal dystrophy: a pathological study. *Arch Ophthalmol* 1964;71:676–682.

24. Thiel HJ, Behnke H: [On the extent of variation of hereditary epithelial corneal dystrophy (Meesmann-Wilke type).] *Ophthalmologica* 1968; 155:81–86.

25. Burns RP: Meesmann's corneal dystrophy. *Trans Am Ophthalmol Soc* 1968;66:530–635.

26. Pülhorn G, Thiel HJ: [Light and electron microscope studies of cyst formation in Meesmann-Wilke hereditary corneal epithelial dystrophy.] *Ophthalmologica* 1974;168:348–359.

27. Fine BS, Yanoff M, Pitts E, et al: Meesmann's epithelial dystrophy of the cornea. *Am J Ophthalmol* 1977;83:633–642.

28. Tremblay M, Dube I: Meesmann's corneal dystrophy: ultrastructural features. *Can J Ophthalmol* 1982;17:24–28.

29. Irvine AD, Corden LD, Swensson O, et al: Mutations in cornea-specific keratins K3 or K12 genes cause Meesmann's corneal dystrophy. *Nat Genet* 1997;16:184–187.

30. Nishida K, Honma Y, Dota A, et al: Isolation and chromosomal localization of a cornea-specific human keratin 12 gene and detection of four mutations in Meesmann corneal epithelial dystrophy. *Am J Hum Genet* 1997;61:1268–1275.

31. Irvine AD, McLean WH: Human keratin diseases: the increasing spectrum of disease and subtlety of the phenotype-genotype correlation. *Br J Dermatol* 1999;140:815–828.

32. Coleman CM, Hannush S, Covello SP, et al: A novel mutation in the helix termination motif of keratin K12 in a US family with Meesmann corneal dystrophy. *Am J Ophthalmol* 1999;128: 687–691.

33. Corden LD, Swensson O, Swensson B, et al: Molecular genetics of Meesmann's corneal dystrophy: ancestral and novel mutations in keratin 12 (K12) and complete sequence of the human KRT12 gene. *Exp Eye Res* 2000;70:41–49.

34. Corden LD, Swensson O, Swensson B, et al: A novel keratin 12 mutation in a German kindred with Meesmann's corneal dystrophy. *Br J Ophthalmol* 2000;84:527–530.

35. Irvine AD, Coleman CM, Moore JE, et al: A novel mutation in KRT12 associated with Meesmann's epithelial corneal dystrophy. *Br J Ophthalmol* 2002;86:729–732.

36. Ku NO, Omary MB: Expression, glycosylation, and phosphorylation of human keratins 8 and 18 in insect cells. *Exp Cell Res* 1994;211: 24–35.

37. Perng MD, Cairns L, van den IJssel P, et al: Intermediate filament interactions can be altered by HSP27 and alphaB-crystallin. *J Cell Sci* 1999;112:2099–2112.

38. van den IJssel P, Norman DG, Quinlan RA: Molecular chaperones: small heat shock proteins in the limelight. *Curr Biol* 1999;9:R103–105.

39. Anton-Lamprecht I, Schnyder UW: Epidermolysis bullosa herpetiformis Dowling-Meara: report of a case and pathomorphogenesis. *Dermatology* 1982;164:221–235.

40. Ishida-Yamamoto A, McGrath JA, Chapman SJ, et al: Epidermolysis bullosa simplex (Dowling-Meara type) is a genetic disease characterized by an abnormal keratin-filament network involving keratins K5 and K14. *J Invest Dermatol* 1991;97:959–968.

41. Holbrook K, Wapner R, Jackson L, et al: Diagnosis and prenatal diagnosis of epidermolysis bullosa herpetiformis (Dowling-Meara) in a mother, two affected children, and an affected fetus. *Prenat Diagn* 1992;12:725–739.

42. Coulombe PA, Hutton ME, Letai A, et al: Point mutations in human keratin 14 genes of epidermolysis bullosa simplex patients: genetic and functional analyses. *Cell* 1991;66:1301–1311.

43. Nakanishi I, Brown SI: Clinicopathologic case report: ultrastructure of the epithelial dystrophy of Meesman. *Arch Ophthalmol* 1975;93: 259–263.

44. Stocker FW, Holt LB: A rare form of hereditary epithelial dystrophy of the cornea: a genetic, clinical and pathological study. *Trans Am Ophthalmol Soc* 1954;52:133–144.

45. Klintworth GK, Sommer JR, Karolak LA, et al: Identification of a new K12 mutation associated with Stocker-Holt corneal dystrophy that differs from mutations found in Meesmann corneal dystrophy. *Invest Ophthalmol Vis Sci* 1999;40(suppl):S563.

46. Lisch W, Steuhl KP, Lisch C, et al: A new, band-shaped and whorled microcystic dystrophy of the corneal epithelium. *Am J Ophthalmol* 1992; 114:35–44.

47. Robin SB, Epstein RJ, Kornmehl EW: Band-shaped, whorled microcystic corneal dystrophy. *Am J Ophthalmol* 1994;117:543–544.

48. Charles NC, Young JA, Kumar A, et al: Band-shaped and whorled microcystic dystrophy of the corneal epithelium. *Ophthalmology* 2000; 107:1761–1764.

49. Bron AJ, Rabinowitz YS: Corneal dystrophies and keratoconus. *Curr Opin Ophthalmol* 1996;7: 71–82.

50. Lisch W, Buttner A, Oeffner F, et al: Lisch corneal dystrophy is genetically distinct from Meesmann corneal dystrophy and maps to xp22.3. *Am J Ophthalmol* 2000;130:461–468.

51. Grayson M, Wilbrandt H: Dystrophy of the anterior limiting membrane of the cornea (Reis-Bücklers type). *Am J Ophthalmol* 1966;61: 345–349.

52. Reis W: [Familial fleck corneal change.] *Dtsch Med Wochenschr* 1917;43:575.

53. Bücklers M: [About a further familial corneal dystrophy (Reis).] *Klin Monatsbl Augenheilkd* 1949;114:386.

54. Thiel HJ, Behnke H: [A hitherto unknown subepithelial hereditary corneal dystrophy.] *Klin Monatsbl Augenheilkd* 1967;150:862–874.

55. Arffa RC: *Grayson's Diseases of the Cornea.* 3rd ed. St Louis: Mosby–Year Book; 1991:372–377.

56. Yamaguchi T, Polack FM, Rowsy JJ: Honeycomb shaped corneal dystrophy: a variation of Reis-Bücklers dystrophy. *Cornea* 1982;1:71.

57. Kanai K, Kaufman HE, Polack FM: Electron microscopic study of Reis-Bücklers' dystrophy. *Ann Ophthalmol* 1973;5:953–962.

58. Griffith DG, Fine BS: Light and electron microscopic observations in a superficial corneal dystrophy probable early Reis-Bücklers' type. *Am J Ophthalmol* 1967;63:1659–1666.

59. Hogan MJ, Wood I: Reis-Bücklers' corneal dystrophy. *Trans Ophthalmol Soc U K* 1971;91: 41–57.

60. Yee RW, Sullivan LS, Lai HT, et al: Linkage mapping of Thiel-Behnke corneal dystrophy (CDB2) to chromosome 10q23-24. *Genomics* 1997;46:152–154.

61. Korvatska E, Munier FL, Chaubert P, et al: On the role of kerato-epithelin in the pathogenesis of 5q31-linked corneal dystrophies. *Invest Ophthalmol Vis Sci* 1999:40:2213–2219.

62. Bernstein HS, Bishop DF, Astrin KH, et al: Fabry disease: six gene rearrangements and an exonic point mutation in the alpha-galactosidase gene. *J Clin Invest* 1989;83:1390–1399.

63. Sher NA, Letson RD, Desnick RJ: The ocular manifestations in Fabry's disease. *Arch Ophthalmol* 1979;97:671–676.

64. Spaeth GL, Frost P: Fabry's disease: its ocular manifestations. *Arch Ophthalmol* 1965; 74:760–769.

65. Siemens HW: Keratosis follicularis spinulosa decalvans. *Arch Dermatol Syphilol* 1926;151: 383–390.

66. Oosterwijk JC, van der Wielen MJ, van de Vosse E, et al: Refinement of the localisation of the X linked keratosis follicularis spinulosa decalvans (KFSD) gene in Xp22.13-p22.2. *J Med Genet* 1995;32:736–739.

67. Christiano AM, Uitto J: Molecular diagnosis of inherited skin diseases: the paradigm of dystrophic epidermolysis bullosa. *Adv Dermatol* 1996;11:199–213.

68. Tong L, Hodgkins PR, Denyer J, et al: The eye in epidermolysis bullosa. *Br J Ophthalmol* 1999;83:323–326.

69. Granek H, Baden HP: Corneal involvement in epidermolysis bullosa simplex. *Arch Ophthalmol* 1980;98:469–472.

70. Stern JK, Lubinsky MS, Durrie DS, et al: Corneal changes, hyperkeratosis, short stature, brachydactyly, and premature birth: a new autosomal dominant syndrome. *Am J Med Genet* 1984; 18:67–77.

71. Blackman HJ, Rodrigues MM, Peck GL: Corneal epithelial lesions in keratosis follicularis (Darier's disease). *Ophthalmology* 1980;87: 931–943.

72. Sakuntabhai A, Ruiz-Perez V, Carter S, et al: Mutations in ATP2A2, encoding a Ca^{2+} pump, cause Darier disease. *Nat Genet* 1999;21:271–277.

73. Witkop CJ Jr, White JG, King RA, et al: Hereditary mucoepithelial dysplasia: a disease apparently of desmosome and gap junction formation. *Am J Hum Genet* 1979;31:414–427.

74. Witkop CJ Jr, White JG, Waring GO: Hereditary mucoepithelial dysplasia, a disease of gap junction and desmosome formation. *Birth Defects* 1982;18:493–511.

75. Berman ER: Diagnosis of metabolic eye disease by chemical analysis of serum, leukocytes and skin fibroblast tissue culture. *Birth Defects* 1976;12:15–51.

76. Rehak A, Selim MM, Yadav G: Richner-Hanhart syndrome (tyrosinaemia-II): report of four cases without ocular involvement. *Br J Dermatol* 1981;104:469–475.

77. Zaleski WA, Hill A, Murray RG: Corneal erosions in tyrosinosis. *Can J Ophthalmol* 1973; 8:556–559.

78. Schermer A, Galvin S, Sun TT: Differentiation-related expression of a major 64K corneal keratin in vivo and in culture suggests limbal location of corneal epithelial stem cells. *J Cell Biol* 1986;103:49–62.

79. Kao WW, Liu CY, Converse RL, et al: Keratin 12–deficient mice have fragile corneal epithelia. *Invest Ophthalmol Vis Sci* 1996;37: 2572–2584.

80. Montgomery RA, Dietz HC: Inhibition of fibrillin 1 expression using U1 snRNA as a vehicle for the presentation of antisense targeting sequence. *Hum Mol Genet* 1997;6:519–525.

81. Millington-Ward S, O'Neill B, Tuohy G, et al: Stratagems in vitro for gene therapies directed to dominant mutations. *Hum Mol Genet* 1997;6:1415–1426.

Stromal Corneal Dystrophies

Nancy L. Flattem, MD, MS

Ming X. Wang, MD, PhD

Anatomically, the group of dystrophies affecting structures immediately posterior to the epithelium, basement membrane, and Bowman's layer are the stromal corneal dystrophies. Stromal dystrophies are divided into two general categories: nonectatic and ectatic. Nonectatic stromal corneal dystrophies include most of the classical anterior stromal corneal dystrophies. These diseases are usually bilateral and genetically inherited, mostly with autosomal dominant transmission. Corneal dystrophies involving primarily the stroma include lattice dystrophy, granular dystrophy, Avellino dystrophy, macular dystrophy, central cloudy dystrophy of François, fleck dystrophy, Schnyder crystalline dystrophy, and gelatinous droplike dystrophy. The ectatic stromal dystrophies are represented in this chapter by keratoconus.

While each of these dystrophies is characterized clinically by a unique set of features under the slit-lamp biomicroscope, and histologically by distinct deposits recognized by special stains, determining a diagnosis can sometimes be difficult because the clinical features overlap. With the advent of molecular genetics and the identification of genes involved in corneal dystrophies, there is now a new level of understanding of the pathogenesis and diagnosis of the stromal corneal dystrophies that may provide new modalities of treatment in the future.

Most stromal dystrophies manifest themselves by 20 years of age, but can be slowly progressive, so patients are often asymptomatic until later in life. The lesions are primarily located in the central part of the cornea, but fleck and macular dystrophies extend to the limbus while lattice corneal dystrophy type II (Meretoja) extends inward from the limbus. The dystrophic deposits lead to the opacification of the cornea, with decreased visual acuity.[1] Chapter 1 discusses the molecular genetics aspect of the stromal dystrophies. This chapter focuses primarily on the clinical manifestations, diagnosis, and management.

3-1

LATTICE CORNEAL DYSTROPHIES

Lattice corneal dystrophies (OMIM 122200) are characterized by bilateral refractile lattice lines in the corneal stroma, particularly anteriorly (Figure 3-1).[2] There are four types of lattice corneal dystrophies[3–7]:

1. Type I (Biber-Haab-Dimmer)
2. Type II (Meretoja) with systemic amyloidosis
3. Type III
4. Type IIIA

Histologically, all lattice types are characterized by deposition of branching "pipestem" lattice figures containing amyloid, which is positive for Congo red staining with apple-green birefringence under polarized light.[7–9] The lattice lines also fluoresce under ultraviolet light.[10] Genetic analysis of patients with lattice corneal dystrophy has identified several DNA point mutations in the *TGFBI* gene encoding keratoepithelin and the gene encoding gelsolin, as discussed in Chapter 1.

3-1-1 Type I

The classic and most common type of lattice corneal dystrophy, type I (Biber-Haab-Dimmer), is the autosomal dominant form that is not associated with systemic amyloidosis.[11] Type I develops at an early age (that is, the teenage years) and is associated with painful bilateral recurrent corneal erosions, often requiring penetrating keratoplasty in the third or fourth decade of life for visual rehabilitation. The delicate branching lattice lines are usually thin and centrally located and are associated with subepithelial opacities and anterior stromal haze.

3-1-2 Type II

Type II (Meretoja syndrome, familial amyloid polyneuropathy type IV, or Finnish type of familial amyloidosis; OMIM 105120) is associated with a systemic amyloidosis, but is a milder corneal dystrophy than type I.[3] Type II has fewer lattice lines, which are more radially oriented and primarily involve the peripheral cornea, sparing the central cornea until later in life, usually when patients are more than 65 years of age. Onset is usually later in life, and significantly fewer visual disturbances are experienced than with type I. In addition, recurrent corneal erosions are rare in type II.

Systemic manifestations include slowly progressive cranial and peripheral neuropathies and dermatologic involvement, including lichen amyloidosis, cutis laxa, blepharochalasis, protruding lips, and mask facies; occasionally, polycythemia vera and ventricular hypertrophy can be found.[12,13] Additional ocular manifestations can include glaucoma and pseudoexfoliation, with or without glaucoma. Like type I, transmission of type II appears to be autosomal dominant. With regard to molecular genetics, the gelsolin gene (on chromosome 9) appears to be the causative gene for lattice type II, rather than the *TGFBI* gene (on chromosome 5), which is implicated in type I.

3-1-3 Types III and IIIA

In contrast to types I and II, an autosomal recessive pattern of inheritance has been observed in families with type III.[4] Lattice corneal dystrophy type III is characterized by thicker lattice lines (Figure 3-2), has a late onset of declining visual acuity (seventh to ninth decade of life), and is not associated with recurrent epithelial erosions.

Unlike type III, which has been found in several Japanese families, type IIIA is found primarily in whites and is often associated with recurrent corneal erosions.[4,6] Also in contrast to type III, type IIIA displays an autosomal dominant inheritance pattern.[6] Like type III, type IIIA also has typically thicker lattice lines, with large amyloid deposits beneath Bowman's layer and midstromally.

3-1-4 Treatment

Treatment of the lattice corneal dystrophies depends on the severity of the symptoms. Recurrent corneal erosions can be managed with the standard therapies of patching, hypertonic agents, artificial tears, or a therapeutic contact lens.[14] With the advent of the excimer laser corneal ablative surgery, phototherapeutic keratectomy (PTK) has been used to treat lattice corneal dystrophy effectively. (The clinical indications and techniques of PTK are discussed in Chapter 6.) Significant visual impairment due to deep stromal scarring needs surgical interventions such as lamellar or penetrating keratoplasty.[7,15] Unfortunately, lattice dystrophy in corneal grafts recurs more frequently than granular or macular corneal dystrophy and can occur in grafts as soon as 3 years after surgery.[14]

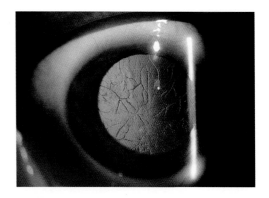

Figure 3-1 *Lattice corneal dystrophy type I. Characteristic lattice lines can be seen in corneal stroma in this retroillumination photograph.*

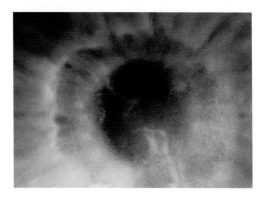

Figure 3-2 *Lattice corneal dystrophy type III. Larger and thicker lattice lines with surrounding opacities can be seen.*

3-2

GRANULAR CORNEAL DYSTROPHIES

Granular corneal dystrophy, also known as *Groenouw I* (OMIM 121900), is an autosomal dominant disorder with at least two predominant clinical phenotypes, the classical and the superficial forms.[16–18] In addition, rare atypical granular dystrophies have been described, including an intermediate form.[19–22] In general, these granular deposits are characterized by grayish white round or snowflake-like opacities in the anterior central stroma (Figure 3-3).[22] Histologically, granular dystrophy is characterized by hyaline deposition that stains positively with Masson trichrome and appears as dense rod-shaped, trapezoidal, or fenestrated bodies on electron microscopy.[17,23,24] Visual impairment usually develops in the fifth decade as the disease progresses, and the corneal stroma between the deposits is generally clear.[22]

3-2-1 Classical Form

The classical form of granular dystrophy is milder than the superficial form and typically has a late onset. The classical granular lesions are characterized by dense white "breadcrumb," annular, or occasionally club-like areas of opacity that are usually small and well demarcated, with clear intervening areas. Individual lesions may resemble snowflakes or popcorn. As the disease progresses, the lesions increase in size and number and possibly coalesce or extend into the deeper and more peripheral stroma. However, the progression is usually slow in classical granular dystrophy, with fewer visual disturbances (usually no earlier than the fifth decade) and less frequent episodes of corneal erosion than the early-onset form. Consequently, there is less need for corneal grafting or other corneal treatments.

3-2-2 Superficial Form

In contrast, the early-onset form of granular dystrophy, the superficial form, presents in the first or second decade of life with confluent subepithelial and superficial opacifications.[22] The clinical course is usually progressive, with an early decrease in vision and frequently recurrent corneal erosions. Management of these patients often requires keratoplasty for visual rehabilitation, as well as therapeutic contact lenses and artificial tears for the recurrent corneal erosions. For severe cases, penetrating keratoplasty has been the traditional surgical approach, but recurrence of the dystrophy is not uncommon.[25–27] Extremely superficial lesions can be treated with epithelial scraping, superficial keratectomy, or lamellar keratoplasty.[18,28] In addition, PTK with the argon fluoride (ArF) excimer laser has been used successfully to ablate superficial deposits in the optical zone and to smooth irregular surfaces.

3-2-3 Molecular Genetics

The classical form of granular dystrophy is primarily associated with the R124H, R124S, and R555W mutations in the *TGFBI* gene, whereas the superficial vari-

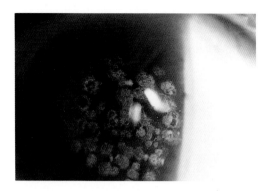

Figure 3-3 *Granular corneal dystrophy. Discrete dense white granular opacities with intervening clear zones characterize this disease.*

ant is associated with the R124L mutation.[29–31] A novel R124L, ΔT125, ΔE126 *TGFBI* mutation was identified in an intermediate form of granular corneal dystrophy.[22] (Chapter 1 contains a detailed discussion of the molecular genetics of granular corneal dystrophy.)

3-3

AVELLINO CORNEAL DYSTROPHY

Avellino corneal dystrophy, also referred to as *combined granular-lattice*, is a variant of granular corneal dystrophy that has features of both lattice and granular corneal dystrophies.[32,33] In addition to the dense white anterior stromal corneal opacities common to granular dystrophies (Figure 3-4A), lattice-like lesions often appear in the mid-to-posterior stroma, as well as opacities occurring in the areas between granular deposits (Figure 3-4B). Typically, the disease progresses from the deposition of granular le-

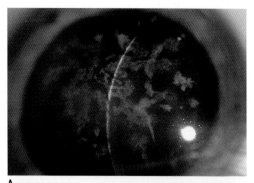

A

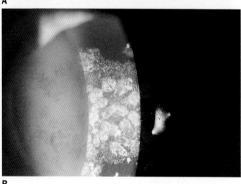

B

Figure 3-4 *Avellino corneal dystrophy. Disease has features of both granular and lattice dystrophies, in that it has both granular and lattice opacities with intervening clear zones. (A) Earlier stage of disease. (B) Advanced stage of disease.*
Courtesy Richard K. Forster, MD, Bascom Palmer Eye Institute, Miami, Florida.

sions first to the development of lattice lesions, with the stromal haze being the last manifestation. All lesions become more prominent with age.

In addition to declining vision, patients also can experience foreign body sensation, pain, and photophobia, which is likely secondary to recurrent corneal erosions. Management for Avellino corneal dystrophy is similar to the treatment for granular and lattice dystrophies, including therapeutic contact lenses and artificial tears for the corneal ulcers and penetrating keratoplasty for the corneal opacifications.

Historically, the name *Avellino* was given to this group of corneal dystrophies because the first reported series of patients was ancestrally linked to the Avellino area in Italy.[32,33] Histologically, the anterior stromal opacities represent both amyloid (as in lattice dystrophy) and hyaline (as in granular dystrophy) properties.[34] A causative DNA point mutation has been identified for Avellino corneal dystrophy in the *TGFBI* gene located on human chromosome 5q31 (R124H),[29] as discussed in detail in Chapter 1.

3-4

MACULAR CORNEAL DYSTROPHY

Macular corneal dystrophy, also known as *Groenouw II* (OMIM 217800), is an autosomal recessive disease that has been linked to human chromosome 16. It is more severe than the granular and lattice forms of corneal dystrophy.[35] The clinical course of macular dystrophy is usually one of progressive visual impairment, which becomes severe by the third and fourth decades of life. In addition, macular dystrophy patients may present with recurrent corneal erosions and attacks of irritation and photophobia that occasionally are quite severe.[36] As early as 3 years of age, a characteristic diffuse fine superficial clouding in the central stroma can be observed, often extending into the peripheral cornea (Figure 3-5A).

As the disease progresses, the gray-white opacities, with indistinct borders and a ground-glass–like haze in the intervening areas, expand to involve the full thickness of the cornea, usually by the second decade of life (Figure 3-5B). The gray-white lesions can even protrude anteriorly to disrupt the corneal surface. Cornea guttata, grayness of Descemet's membrane, and deep posterior focal plaques in the periphery can also be observed. Frequently associated with macular dystrophy is reduced central corneal thickness. Histologically, the deposits are located throughout the corneal stroma, intracellularly and extracellularly, and stain positively with colloidal iron or Alcian blue, representing mucopolysaccharides.[23,37]

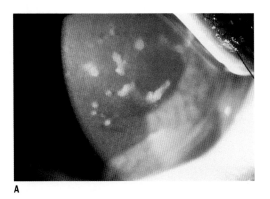

A

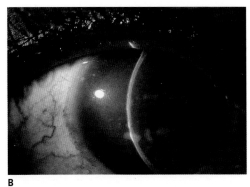

B

Management of macular corneal dystrophy is tailored to the patient, but could include the standard treatment for recurrent corneal erosions (therapeutic contact lenses or hypertonic agents), tinted cosmetic lenses for photophobia, PTK for early stages of the disease, lamellar keratoplasty, or, most commonly, penetrating keratoplasty. Notably, recurrences in the grafts are not common in macular corneal dystrophy.

Macular corneal dystrophy has been divided into two types, according to antigenic keratan sulfate (AgKS) immunoreactivity.[38] AgKS immunoreactivity is absent in both corneal tissue and serum in type I, whereas type II has detectable and often normal serum AgKS levels, but has corneal accumulations that react with a monoclonal anti–keratan sulfate (KS) antibody.[38] In addition, a type IA, described in families from Saudi Arabia, is characterized by an absence of both serum and corneal stroma AgKS immunoreactivity but anti–KS antibody–reactive accumulations within keratocytes.[39] Keratan sulfate proteoglycans, as the name indicates, are sulfated in the normal cornea and, without proper addition of sulfate

Figure 3-5 *Macular corneal dystrophy. Disease is characterized by anterior and deep stromal opacities with indistinct borders; lesions sometimes extend out to corneal periphery. (A) Earlier stage of disease. (B) Advanced stage of disease.*
Courtesy Richard K. Forster, MD, Bascom Palmer Eye Institute, Miami, Florida. Part A reproduced with permission from Parrish RK II, ed: The University of Miami Bascom Palmer Eye Institute Atlas of Ophthalmology. *Philadelphia: Current Medicine, Inc.; 2000.*

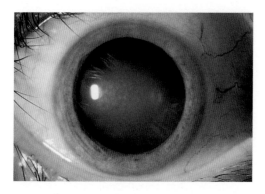

Figure 3-6 *Central cloudy dystrophy of François.*

groups, deposits will form in the corneal stroma in type I.[40] Mutations have been identified in the carbohydrate sulphotransferase gene (*CHST6*) encoding corneal *N*-acetylglucosamine-6-sulphotransferase (C-GlcNAc6ST) that likely play an important role in the pathophysiology of the disease,[41] as discussed in Chapter 1.

3-5

CENTRAL CLOUDY DYSTROPHY OF FRANÇOIS

Central cloudy dystrophy of François is a relatively common disease. The inheritance pattern is often autosomal dominant. The disease typically involves the central posterior corneal stroma bilaterally.[42] Small and often polygonal patches of grayish opacities are seen, with a posterior mosaic or crocodile pattern (Figure 3-6). The clinical presentation of the disease closely resembles that of posterior crocodile shagreen, except that the latter typically is not genetically inherited and more commonly has peripheral and anterior stromal lesions.[43,44] Patients with central cloudy dystrophy of François typically do not have a history of recurrent corneal erosion, as in other anterior stromal dystrophies, because the disease does not involve epithelial or endothelial cell dysfunction, as is true for lattice dystrophy for example. Histopathologically, it is believed that the dystrophic material contains mucopolysaccharide and lipid-like substances. The disease is rarely progressive and, since vision is not usually affected, no treatment is needed.

3-6

FLECK DYSTROPHY

Fleck dystrophy, also known as *François-Neetens dystrophy* (OMIM 121850), *speckled dystrophy*, or *mouchetée dystrophy*, is a rarely recognized autosomal dominant disease that can be present at birth.[45] Characteristic findings include small oval, stellate, comma-shaped, or doughnut-shaped opacities in the anterior corneal stroma, with clear intervening areas (Figure 3-7). The fine granular flecks can involve the central or peripheral cornea or both and the entire stroma, except Bowman's layer.[46] The tiny lesions, with discrete or scalloped borders, may be best appreciated on retroillumination and may appear refractile.[47] Punctate cortical lens opacities can also be observed.[48] Vision is generally not affected, and there is little progression of the disease.[49] Some patients complain of photophobia, and some may have decreased corneal sensation. Histologically, the lesion appears to be aggregated, and distended keratocytes contain glycosaminoglycans, as demonstrated with Alcian blue or colloidal iron stains. Because patients are asymptomatic, treatment is not indicated.

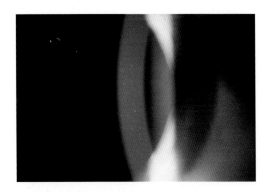

Figure 3-7 *Fleck dystrophy. Note discrete small comma-shaped and oval anterior stromal opacities.*
Courtesy Richard K. Forster, MD, Bascom Palmer Eye Institute, Miami, Florida. Reproduced with permission from Parrish RK II, ed: The University of Miami Bascom Palmer Eye Institute Atlas of Ophthalmology. *Philadelphia: Current Medicine, Inc.; 2000.*

3-7

SCHNYDER CRYSTALLINE DYSTROPHY

Schnyder crystalline dystrophy (OMIM 121900), also called *central crystalline dystrophy of Schnyder*, is a rare autosomal dominant

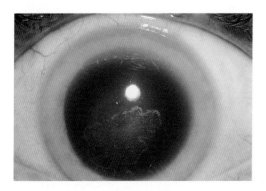

Figure 3-8 *Schnyder crystalline dystrophy. Polychromatic fine crystals can be seen in disciform pattern in anterior corneal stroma.*
Courtesy Richard K. Forster, MD, Bascom Palmer Eye Institute, Miami, Florida. Reproduced with permission from Parrish RK II, ed: The University of Miami Bascom Palmer Eye Institute Atlas of Ophthalmology. *Philadelphia: Current Medicine, Inc.; 2000.*

disease. Clinically, polychromatic fine crystals can be seen in disciform, geographic, or annular patterns in the anterior corneal stroma and occasionally extend into the deeper stromal layers (Figure 3-8).[50] The intervening stromal areas are usually clear, but occasionally small diffuse opaque punctate lesions can be seen, and even a progressive diffuse stromal haze can be observed in some individuals.[51–53] Sometimes, patients may experience a progressive decline in sensation in the cornea overlying the lesions, but corneal erosions are rare. While the crystalline lesions are often centrally located, vision is usually not significantly affected and the disease infrequently progresses.

Histologically, Schnyder dystrophy is characterized by cholesterol crystals and lipid and neutral globular fat deposition.[50,54–60] Additional findings can include systemic hyperlipidemia and arcus senilis or arcus lipoides in the peripheral cornea. Therefore, included in the management of these patients should be fasting blood levels of cholesterol and triglyceride and lipoprotein electrophoresis. The ocular symptoms should be treated when they become significant. Lamellar or penetrating grafts may be needed if the decline in acuity and corneal sensation becomes severe. As would be expected by the cause of the disease, cholesterol crystals do recur.[59] The use of the excimer laser in treating the anterior stromal opacities of this disease is still experimental, but may prove to be a valuable therapy.

3-8

GELATINOUS DROP-LIKE CORNEAL DYSTROPHY

Gelatinous drop-like corneal dystrophy, also called *familial subepithelial amyloidosis* (OMIM 204870), is a rare autosomal recessive familial corneal amyloidosis predominantly affecting Japanese people.[61] The lesions of gelatinous drop-like corneal dystrophy are opaque on direct illumination and translucent on retroillumination. The characteristic lesions that give the cornea a mulberry-like appearance are multiple subepithelial gelatinous excrescences (Figure 3-9) that appear early in life, usually between the ages of 8 and 18.[62]

As the disease progresses, the patient experiences photophobia, lacrimation, foreign body sensation, and declining vision. Neovascularization often accompanies advanced disease. Histologic studies reveal large amyloid-staining deposits in the subepithelial and anterior stromal regions, with disruption of Bowman's layer. While the overlying epithelium may be hyperplastic or atrophic, the posterior stroma, Descemet's membrane, and the endothelium are usually normal.[62,63]

Treatment of advanced disease includes superficial keratectomy, lamellar keratoplasty, and penetrating keratoplasty. Because recurrence of the disease approaches 50% of eyes after penetrating keratoplasty, limbal allografting is being performed in the attempt to diminish the likelihood of recurrence.[64] DNA mutations have been identified in the *M1S1* gene on chromosome 1p31 (discussed in Chapter 1), and further study of the molecular pathophysiology may shed light on the cause of the disease and help identify better modalities of treatment.

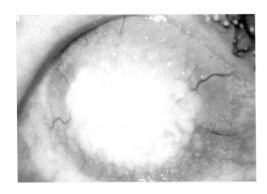

Figure 3-9 *Gelatinous drop-like dystrophy. Opaque gelatinous drop-like corneal opacities can be seen. Characteristic lesions that give cornea mulberry-like appearance are multiple subepithelial gelatinous excrescences.*

Reproduced with permission from External Disease and Cornea, *Section 8 of the Basic and Clinical Science Course. San Francisco: American Academy of Ophthalmology; 2002–2003.*

KERATOCONUS

Keratoconus represents one of the most common clinical indications for penetrating keratoplasty. The disease is characterized by progressive thinning and forward ectasia of the cornea. About 10% of patients have a family history of the condition, and the transmission pattern can be autosomal dominant or recessive. Keratoconus is often associated with systemic diseases such as Down syndrome, atopic disease,[65] vernal catarrh,[66] retinitis pigmentosa,[67] aniridia, retinopathy of prematurity,[68] Marfan syndrome,[69] and Ehlers-Danlos syndrome.[70]

Typically, the disease has an onset in young adulthood and some patients have a history of rubbing the eye or wearing hard contact lenses. The disease appears to have two general types: a severe, rapidly progressive type, which often requires keratoplasty before age 30; and a mild-to-moderate, slowly progressive type, in which patients can maintain functional vision with nonsurgical correction such as rigid gas-permeable lenses or spectacles.

Keratoconus is characterized by a group of diagnostic signs, including: coned appearance of the cornea seen on external examination (Figure 3-10A); iron line, or Fleischer ring (Figure 3-10B), surrounding the base of the cone; vertical stress lines in deep corneal stroma, or Vogt's striae (Figure 3-10C); central and inferior stromal thinning (Figure 3-10D). With disease progression, Descemet's membrane can rupture and aqueous can expand into the corneal stroma, causing significant edema, or hydrops (Figure 3-10E), which may later heal and result in anterior stromal scarring (Figure 3-10F).

Histopathologically, Bowman's layer and epithelial basement membrane are found to be fragmented, and activated keratocytes and fibrotic tissue are seen in the diseased areas.[71] Abnormal proteoglycan material is seen in the stroma.[72] With hydrops, a break in Descemet's membrane is seen and the remaining endothelial cells migrate and stretch to cover the exposed area of corneal stroma.

The molecular cause of keratoconus is still uncertain. A number of investigators have found biochemical and cellular abnormalities in keratoconus corneas, suggesting the future direction of research to identify the primary pathologic event. These findings include increased collagen cross-linking in keratoconus corneas,[73] reduced protein content,[74] reduced RNA metabolism in cultured stromal cells from keratoconus patients,[75] abnormal proteoglycan metabolism,[76] abnormalities in the glycoproteins on the surface of the keratocytes,[77] reduced amount of keratan sulfate,[78] and abnormal location and structural relationship between proteoglycan and collagen fibrils.[79] In addition to these biochemical and structural ab-

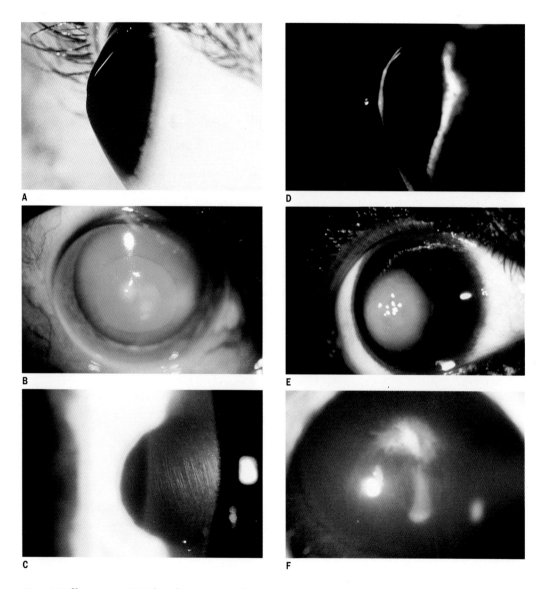

Figure 3-10 *Keratoconus. (A) Coned appearance of cornea seen on external examination. (B) Iron line (Fleischer ring) surrounding base of cone. (C) Vertical stress lines in deep corneal stroma (Vogt's striae). (D) Central and inferior stromal thinning. (E) Hydrops. (F) Late-stage anterior stromal scar.*
Courtesy Resident Slide Collection, Wills Eye Hospital, 1991.

normalities, degradative enzymes have also been found to be increased in keratoconus corneas, including collagenase,[80] gelatinase,[81] and lysosomal acid hydrolase,[82] as well as a reduced level of alpha-1-proteinase inhibitor.[83] Taking these findings together, it seems plausible that keratoconus may be caused by some primary structural abnormalities and interaction in collagen fibrils and proteoglycans, coupled with an increased level of degradative enzymes, weakening the biomechanical strength of the cornea.

The treatment of keratoconus consists of medical treatment with a rigid gas-permeable lens to correct the high amount of regular and irregular astigmatism. More than 80% of patients do not require keratoplasty.[84] An acute episode of hydrops is usually treated conservatively, as it typically heals. PTK with the excimer laser is an effective treatment to remove anterior stromal scarring and to smooth the tip of the cone and improve contact lens tolerance, although caution must be exercised regarding the depth of the treatment in these thin corneas. Corneal transplantation remains the most effective treatment for advanced disease. Lamellar keratoplasty is no longer popular because of surgical difficulty and unsatisfactory visual outcome; penetrating keratoplasty is the treatment of choice. The prognosis of penetrating keratoplasty for keratoconus is excellent, with greater than 80% of grafts maintaining 20/40 or better vision.[85,86] The postkeratoplasty residual astigmatism and myopic refractive error can be effectively managed by laser-assisted in situ keratomileusis (LASIK).[87]

3-10

CONCLUSION

The nonectatic stromal corneal dystrophies represent a collection of corneal dystrophic conditions that have been divided into specific categories based on clinical and histologic characteristics. Although there is some degree of overlap in their clinical features, the identification of specific causative genes associated with these anterior stromal dystrophies not only has improved the accuracy of diagnosis, but also is shedding new light on the pathogenesis of this group of dystrophic diseases.[88–91] In addition to conservative medical management, stromal corneal dystrophies can now be effectively treated with excimer laser PTK, improving the chance of avoiding penetrating keratoplasty in many patients. The treatment of choice for ectatic corneal dystrophy, as represented by keratoconus, is still the rigid gas-permeable lens and, in advanced stages, penetrating keratoplasty. The primary molecular events that give rise to keratoconus have yet to be elucidated, despite intensive studies of biochemical and structural abnormalities in this disease.

REFERENCES

1. Van den Berg TJ, Hwan BS, Delleman JW: The intraocular straylight function in some hereditary corneal dystrophies. *Doc Ophthalmol* 1993;85:13–19.

2. McKusick VA: *Online Mendelian Inheritance in Man* (OMIM). Center for Medical Genetics, Johns Hopkins University, and National Center for Biotechnology Information, National Library of Medicine, 2002. www.ncbi.nlm.nih.gov/omim

3. Meretoja J: Comparative histopathological and clinical findings in eyes with lattice corneal dystrophy of two different types. *Ophthalmologica* 1972;165:15–37.

4. Hida T, Proia AD, Kigasawa K, et al: Histopathologic and immunochemical features of lattice corneal dystrophy type III. *Am J Ophthalmol* 1987;104:249–254.

5. Hida T, Tsubota K, Kigasawa K, et al: Clinical features of a newly recognized type of lattice corneal dystrophy. *Am J Ophthalmol* 1987;104: 241–248.

6. Stock EL, Feder RS, O'Grady RB, et al: Lattice corneal dystrophy type IIIA: clinical and histopathologic correlations. *Arch Ophthalmol* 1991;109:354–358.

7. Klintworth GK, Ferry AP, Sugar A, et al: Recurrence of lattice corneal dystrophy type 1 in the corneal grafts of two siblings. *Am J Ophthalmol* 1982;94:540–546.

8. Klintworth GK: Lattice corneal dystrophy: an inherited variety of amyloidosis restricted to the cornea. *Am J Pathol* 1967;50:371–399.

9. Schmitt-Bernard CF, Guittard C, Arnaud B, et al: BIGH3 exon 14 mutations lead to intermediate type I/IIIA of lattice corneal dystrophies. *Invest Ophthalmol Vis Sci* 2000;41:1302–1308.

10. Dark AJ, Thompson DS: Lattice dystrophy of the cornea: a clinical and microscopic study. *Br J Ophthalmol* 1960;44:257.

11. Gorevic PD, Rodrigues MM, Krachmer JH, et al: Lack of evidence for protein AA reactivity in amyloid deposits of lattice corneal dystrophy and amyloid corneal degeneration. *Am J Ophthalmol* 1984;98:216–224.

12. Meretoja J: Familial systemic paramyloidosis with lattice dystrophy of the cornea, progressive cranial neuropathy, skin changes and various internal symptoms: a previously unrecognized heritable syndrome. *Ann Clin Res* 1969;1:314–324.

13. Starck T, Kenyon KR, Hanninen LA, et al: Clinical and histopathologic studies of two families with lattice corneal dystrophy and familial systemic amyloidosis (Meretoja syndrome). *Ophthalmology* 1991;98:1197–1206.

14. Mannis MJ, De Sousa LB, Gross RH: The stromal dystrophies. In: Krachmer JH, Mannis MJ, Holland EJ, eds: *Cornea and External Disease: Clinical Diagnosis and Management*. St Louis: CV Mosby Co; 1997:1043–1062.

15. Meisler DM, Fine M: Recurrence of clinical signs of lattice corneal dystrophy (type I) in corneal transplants. *Am J Ophthalmol* 1984;97: 210–214.

16. Rodrigues MM, Gaster RN, Pratt MV: Unusual superficial confluent form of granular corneal dystrophy. *Ophthalmology* 1983;90: 1507–1511.

17. Møller HU: Inter-familial variability and intra-familial similarities of granular corneal dystrophy Groenouw type I with respect to biomicroscopical appearance and symptomatology. *Acta Ophthalmol (Copenh)* 1989;67:669–677.

18. Sajjadi SH, Javadi MA: Superficial juvenile granular dystrophy. *Ophthalmology* 1992;99: 95–102.

19. Fujiki K, Hotta Y, Nakayasu K, et al: Homozygotic patient with betaig-h3 gene mutation in granular dystrophy. *Cornea* 1998;17:288–292.

20. Okada M, Yamamoto S, Watanabe H, et al: Granular corneal dystrophy with homozygous mutations in the kerato-epithelin gene. *Am J Ophthalmol* 1998;126:169–176.

21. Okada M, Yamamoto S, Inoue Y, et al: Severe corneal dystrophy phenotype caused by homozygous R124H keratoepithelin mutations. *Invest Ophthalmol Vis Sci* 1998;39:1947–1953.

22. Dighiero P, Drunat S, D'Hermies F, et al: A novel variant of granular corneal dystrophy caused by association of 2 mutations in the TGFBI gene—R124L and DeltaT125-DeltaE126. *Arch Ophthalmol* 2000;118:814–818.

23. Jones ST, Zimmerman LE: Histopathologic differentiation of granular, macular, and lattice dystrophies of the cornea. *Am J Ophthalmol* 1961; 51:394–410.

24. Akiya S, Brown SI: Granular dystrophy of the cornea: characteristic electron microscopic lesion. *Arch Ophthalmol* 1970;84:179–192.

25. Rodrigues MM, McGavic JS: Recurrent corneal granular dystrophy: a clinicopathologic study. *Trans Am Ophthalmol Soc* 1975;73:306–316.

26. Johnson BL, Brown SI, Zaidman GW: A light and electron microscopic study of recurrent granular dystrophy of the cornea. *Am J Ophthalmol* 1981;92:49–58.

27. Ruusuvaara P, Setala K, Tarkkanen A: Granular corneal dystrophy with early stromal manifestation: a clinical and electron microscopical study. *Acta Ophthalmol Scand* 1990;68:525–531.

28. Lyons CJ, McCartney AC, Kirkness CM, et al: Granular corneal dystrophy: visual results and pattern of recurrence after lamellar or penetrating keratoplasty. *Ophthalmology* 1994;101: 1812–1817.

29. Munier FL, Korvatska E, Djemai A, et al: Kerato-epithelin mutations in four 5q31-linked corneal dystrophies. *Nat Genet* 1997;15:247–251.

30. Korvatska E, Munier FL, Djemai A, et al: Mutation hot spots in 5q31-linked corneal dystrophies. *Am J Hum Genet* 1998;62:320–324.

31. Mashima Y, Nakamura Y, Noda K, et al: A novel mutation at codon 124 (R124L) in the BIGH3 gene is associated with a superficial variant of granular corneal dystrophy. *Arch Ophthalmol* 1999;117:90–93.

32. Folberg R, Alfonso E, Croxatto JO, et al: Clinically atypical granular corneal dystrophy with pathologic features of lattice-like amyloid deposits: a study of three families. *Ophthalmology* 1988;95:46–51.

33. Holland EJ, Daya SM, Stone EM, et al: Avellino corneal dystrophy: clinical manifestations and natural history. *Ophthalmology* 1992; 99:1564–1568.

34. Folberg R, Stone EM, Sheffield VC, et al: The relationship between granular, lattice type 1, and Avellino corneal dystrophies: a histopathologic study. *Arch Ophthalmol* 1994;112: 1080–1085.

35. Vance JM, Jonasson F, Lennon F, et al: Linkage of a gene for macular corneal dystrophy to chromosome 16. *Am J Hum Genet* 1996;58: 757–762.

36. Jonasson F, Johannsson JH, Garner A, et al: Macular corneal dystrophy in Iceland. *Eye* 1989; 3:446–454.

37. Jones ST, Zimmerman LE: Macular dystrophy of the cornea (Groenouw type II). *Am J Ophthalmol* 1959;47:1–16.

38. Yang CJ, SundarRaj N, Thonar EJ, et al: Immunohistochemical evidence of heterogeneity in macular corneal dystrophy. *Am J Ophthalmol* 1988;106:65–71.

39. Klintworth GK, Oshima E, al-Rajhi A, et al: Macular corneal dystrophy in Saudi Arabia: a study of 56 cases and recognition of a new immunophenotype. *Am J Ophthalmol* 1997;124: 9–18.

40. Lewis D, Davies Y, Nieduszynski IA, et al: Ultrastructural localization of sulfated and unsulfated keratan sulfate in normal and macular corneal dystrophy type I. *Glycobiology* 2000;10: 305–312.

41. Akama TO, Nishida K, Nakayama J, et al: Macular corneal dystrophy type I and type II are caused by distinct mutations in a new sulphotransferase gene. *Nat Genet* 2000;26:237–241.

42. François J: [A new hereditary dystrophy of the cornea.] *J Genet Hum* 1956;5:189–196.

43. Goodside V: Posterior crocodile shagreen. *Am J Ophthalmol* 1958;46:748–750.

44. Krachmer JH, Dubord PJ, Rodrigues MM, et al: Corneal posterior crocodile shagreen and polymorphic amyloid degeneration. *Arch Ophthalmol* 1983;101:54–59.

45. François J, Neetens A: [New hereditary dystrophy of the corneal parenchyma (fleck hereditary dystrophy).] *Bull Soc Belge Ophtalmol* 1957; 114:641–646.

46. Stankovic, I, Stankovic D: [The fleck hereditary dystrophy of the corneal parenchyma.] *Ann Ocul (Paris)* 1964;1997:52–57.

47. Waring GO III, Rodrigues MM, Laibson PR: Corneal dystrophies, I: dystrophies of the epithelium, Bowman's layer and stroma. *Surv Ophthalmol* 1978;23:71–122.

48. Purcell JJ Jr, Krachmer JH, Weingeist TA: Fleck corneal dystrophy. *Arch Ophthalmol* 1977; 95:440–444.

49. Birndorf LA, Ginsberg SP: Hereditary fleck dystrophy associated with decreased corneal sensitivity. *Am J Ophthalmol* 1972;73:670–672.

50. Bron AJ, Williams HP, Carruthers ME: Hereditary crystalline stromal dystrophy of Schnyder, I: clinical features of a family with hyperlipoproteinaemia. *Br J Ophthalmol* 1972; 56:383–399.

51. Luxenberg M: Hereditary crystalline dystrophy of the cornea. *Am J Ophthalmol* 1967;63: 507–511.

52. Ehlers N, Mathiessen ME: Hereditary crystalline corneal dystrophy of Schnyder. *Acta Ophthalmologica* 1973; 51:316–324.

53. Weiss JS: Schnyder's dystrophy of the cornea: a Swede–Finn connection. *Cornea* 1992;1: 93–101.

54. Rodrigues MM, Kruth HS, Krachmer JH, et al: Unesterified cholesterol in Schnyder's corneal crystalline dystrophy. *Am J Ophthalmol* 1987;104: 157–163.

55. Freddo TF, Polack FM, Leibowitz HM: Ultrastructural changes in the posterior layers of the cornea in Schnyder's crystalline dystrophy. *Cornea* 1989;8:170–177.

56. Weiss JS, Rodrigues M, Rajagopalan S, et al: Atypical Schnyder's crystalline dystrophy of the cornea: a light and electron microscopic study. *Proc Int Soc Eye Res* 1990;6:198.

57. Weiss JS, Rodrigues M, Rajagopalan S, et al: Schnyder's corneal dystrophy: clinical, ultrastructural, and histochemical studies. *Ophthalmology* 1990;97(suppl):141.

58. Weller RO, Rodger FC: Crystalline stromal dystrophy: histochemistry and ultrastructure of the cornea. *Br J Ophthalmol* 1980;64:46–52.

59. Garner A, Tripathi RC: Hereditary crystalline stromal dystrophy of Schnyder, II: histopathology and ultrastructure. *Br J Ophthalmol* 1972;56:400–408.

60. Rodrigues MM, Kruth HS, Krachmer JH, et al: Cholesterol localization in ultrathin frozen sections in Schnyder's corneal crystalline dystrophy. *Am J Ophthalmol* 1990;110:513–517.

61. Shindo S: Gelatinous drop-like corneal dystrophy: case report with histopathological findings. *Jpn J Clin Ophthalmol* 1969;23:1167.

62. Gartry DS, Falcon MG, Cox RW: Primary gelatinous drop-like keratopathy. *Br J Ophthalmol* 1989;73:661–664.

63. Ohinishi Y, Shinoda Y, Ishibashi T, et al: The origin of amyloid in gelatinous drop-like corneal dystrophy. *Curr Eye Res* 1982–1983;2:225–231.

64. Toshida H, Uesugi Y, Nakayasu K, et al: Keratoplasty for gelatinous drop-like corneal dystrophy. *Jpn J Clin Ophthalmol* 1995;49:449.

65. Spencer WH, Fisher JJ: The association of keratoconus with atopic dermatitis. *Am J Ophthalmol* 1959;47:332.

66. Copeman PW: Eczema and keratoconus. *Br Med J* 1965;5468:977–979.

67. Streiff EB: [Keratoconus and pigmentary retinopathy.] *Bull Mem Soc Fr Ophtalmol* 1952; 65:323.

68. Lorfel RS, Sugar HS: Keratoconus associated with retrolental fibroplasia. *Ann Ophthalmol* 1976; 8:449–450.

69. Austin MG, Schaefer RF: Marfan syndrome with unusual blood vessel manifestations: primary medionecrosis, dissection of the right innominate. *Arch Pathol Lab Med* 1957;64:205.

70. Judisch GF, Waziri M, Krachmer JH: Ocular Ehlers-Danlos syndrome with normal lysyl hydroxylase activity. *Arch Ophthalmol* 1976;94: 1489–1491.

71. Pataa C, Joyone L, Roucher F: [Ultrastructure of keratoconus.] *Arch Ophtalmol (Paris)* 1970; 30:403–417.

72. Gottinger W, Aubock L: [Electron-microscopic findings in keratoconus.] *Klin Monatsbl Augenheilkd* 1970;157:762–772.

73. Cannon DJ, Foster CS: Collagen crosslinking in keratoconus. *Invest Ophthalmol Vis Sci* 1978;17:63–65.

74. Critchfield JW, Calandra AJ, Nesburn AB, et al: Keratoconus, I: biochemical studies. *Exp Eye Res* 1988;46:953–963.

75. Yue BY, Sugar J, Benveniste K: RNA metabolism in cultures of corneal stromal cells from patients with keratoconus. *Proc Soc Exp Biol Med* 1985;178:126–132.

76. Bleckmann H, Kresse H: Studies on the glycosaminoglycan metabolism of cultured fibroblasts from human keratoconus corneas. *Exp Eye Res* 1980;30:215–219.

77. Yue BY, Panjwani N, Sugar J, et al: Glyco-conjugate abnormalities in cultured kerato-conus stromal cells. *Arch Ophthalmol* 1988;106: 1709–1712.

78. Funderburgh JL, Funderburgh ML, Rodrigues MM, et al: Altered antigenicity of keratan sulfate proteoglycan in selected corneal diseases. *Invest Ophthalmol Vis Sci* 1990;31:419–428.

79. Meek KM, Elliott GF, Gyi TJ, et al: The structure of normal and keratoconus human corneas. *Ophthalmic Res* 1987;19:6.

80. Ihalainen A, Salo T, Forsius H, et al: Increase in type I and type IV collagenolytic activity in primary cultures of keratoconus cornea. *Eur J Clin Invest* 1986;16:78–84.

81. Kenney MC, Chwa M, Escobar M, et al: Altered gelatinolytic activity by keratoconus corneal cells. *Biochem Biophys Res Commun* 1989; 161:353–357.

82. Sawaguchi S, Yue BY, Sugar J, et al: Lysosomal enzyme abnormalities in keratoconus. *Arch Ophthalmol* 1989;107:1507–1510.

83. Sawaguchi S, Twining SS, Yue BY, et al: Alpha-1 proteinase inhibitor levels in keratoconus. *Exp Eye Res* 1990;50:549–554.

84. Kennedy RH, Bourne WM, Dyer JA: A 48-year clinical and epidemiologic study of keratoconus. *Am J Ophthalmol* 1986;101:267–273.

85. Payne JW: Primary penetrating keratoplasty for keratoconus: a long-term follow-up. *Cornea* 1982;1:21.

86. Paglen PG, Fine M, Abbott RL, et al: The prognosis for keratoplasty in keratoconus. *Ophthalmology* 1982;89:651–654.

87. Tran UL, Kagan O, Yang HM, et al: Preoperative predictive factors influencing the clinical outcome of LASIK after penetrating keratoplasty. *Invest Ophthalmol Vis Sci* 2002;43:B120.

88. Wang MX, Forster RK: Dystrophies, degenerations, and congenital anomalies of the cornea. In: Parrish RK II, ed: *The University of Miami Bascom Palmer Eye Institute Atlas of Ophthalmology*. Philadelphia: Current Medicine, Inc.; 2000;1: 91–98.

89. Wang MX, Munier FL, Yang R, et al: Molecular basis of lattice corneal dystrophies. *Invest Ophthalmol Vis Sci* 1998;39(suppl):S1.

90. Wang MX, Munier FL, Araki-Saski, et al: TGFBI gene transcript is transforming growth factor-beta–responsive and cell density–dependent in a human corneal epithelial cell line. *Ophthalmic Genet* 2002 (in press).

91. Munier FL, Frueh BE, Othenin-Girard P, et al: BIGH3 mutation spectrum in corneal dystrophies. *Invest Ophthalmol Vis Sci* 2002;43: 949–954.

CHAPTER 4

Endothelial Corneal Dystrophies

Rajy M. Rouweyha, MD
Richard W. Yee, MD

From an anatomic standpoint, the endothelial dystrophies represent those of the most posterior portion of the cornea. These dystrophies include Fuchs endothelial dystrophy, congenital hereditary endothelial dystrophy, posterior polymorphous dystrophy, and iridocorneal endothelial syndrome. Molecular genetics studies in recent years have begun to reveal the genetic loci and possible candidate genes involved in dystrophies of the corneal endothelium.

4-1

ENDOTHELIAL PHYSIOLOGY

The endothelium, a single layer of flat hexagonal cells that forms a continuous mosaic, lies posteriorly on Descemet's membrane. The endothelial cell layer is derived from embryonic neural crest cells and is greatly responsible for maintaining corneal transparency. Endothelial cells pump out excess water from the stroma of the cornea, thereby allowing collagen fibrils of the stroma to remain at a fixed spacing from each other. These cells exhibit great metabolic activity, as indicated by the presence of numerous large mitochondria, consistent with a high energy demand for cellular processes (for example, active ion transport).

Endothelial cells do not possess any significant mitotic activity after birth. They continue to die and decrease throughout life (endothelial cell apoptosis), resulting in a gradual decrease of endothelial cell population with age. The cell density decreases from approximately 4000 cells/mm^2 at birth to 2000 cells/mm^2 by the ninth decade of life. As cell death occurs, neighboring cells expand to cover the vacant area. The endothelial cell layer is capable of preserving function despite significant cell loss via tremendous enlargement. Generally, the endothelium can still maintain corneal function at cell densities below 800 cells/mm^2.

The corneal endothelium is a leaky cell layer that has markedly higher water permeability than the corneal epithelium. The greater water permeability is necessary for the nutrition of stromal and epithelial cells, as the cornea is an avascular structure, and diffusion from the limbal blood vessels would be insufficient to meet the demands of the central cornea.[1] This excess water, however, must be removed to prevent stromal edema.

The corneal endothelium maintains corneal transparency by transferring water from its basal to apical surface against a pressure gradient equivalent to the intraocular pressure (IOP). The maintenance of corneal transparency is actually an active process requiring metabolic energy. This endothelial ion transporter is believed to be a Na^+/K^+-ATPase (sodium/potassium-adenosinetriphosphatase) pump located on the basolateral membrane. Thus, the endothelium, often referred to as a *fluid pump*, does not actually pump water directly out of the stroma. Rather, it utilizes the mechanism of active transport of ions from the stroma into the aqueous, with passive secondary movement of water.

The control of stromal hydration is much more complex than the active transport of ions by the endothelium. There is also a significant contribution from the epithelial cell layer. The different mechanisms responsible for the control of stromal hydration include epithelial and endothelial barrier function, swelling pressure of the stroma, ion transport by the epithelium and endothelium, IOP, and corneal surface evaporation. The greatest contribution to the control of stromal hydration is achieved by the corneal endothelium. Any disorder that compromises the endothelium to a sufficient extent will result in corneal edema. The endothelial corneal dystrophies—Fuchs endothelial dystrophy, congenital hereditary endothelial dystrophy, and posterior polymorphous dystrophy—are all inherited conditions of the corneal endothelium that can result clinically in corneal clouding and loss of visual acuity.

4-2

FUCHS ENDOTHELIAL DYSTROPHY

In 1910, Ernst Fuchs, a German ophthalmologist, reported 13 cases of bilateral central corneal clouding, epithelial edema, and impaired corneal sensitivity in elderly patients.[2] It wasn't until 1916 that Leonhard Koeppe described endothelial dellen.[3] In 1921, Alfred Vogt coined the term *guttae* (plural of the Latin *gutta*, meaning "droplet") to describe corneas containing multiple drop-like endothelial excrescences.[4] Kirby and Gifford confirmed the predominant role of the endothelium in 1925.[5] Despite the significant contribution from others after Fuchs' initial description of the entity, this endothelial dystrophy is named after him, as he was the first to describe its salient features.

The disease is caused by a pleomorphic dysfunctional endothelium and an abnormal basement membrane. The earliest sign, corneal guttae (hyaline excrescences on Descemet's membrane), can progress to stromal edema, epithelial bullae, and subepithelial fibrosis (or scarring). This entity is a bilateral, but often asymmetric posterior corneal dystrophy that usually manifests after the fourth decade of life. It is one of the most common corneal dystrophies in the United States.

4-2-1 Genetics and Causation

The condition appears to have an inherited predisposition (although often a positive family history is lacking) and is transmitted in an autosomal dominant fashion, with greater expressivity in females. The chromosomal abnormality and genetic locus responsible for Fuchs dystrophy have yet to be determined, although evidence exists

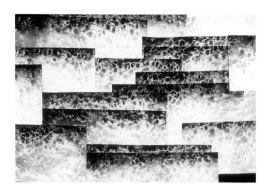

Figure 4-1 *Fuchs endothelial dystrophy. Specular microscopic montage showing guttae.*

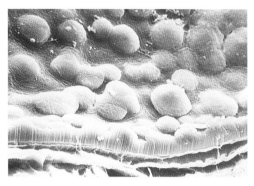

Figure 4-2 *Fuchs endothelial dystrophy. Scanning electron microscopy showing excrescences.*

that the *COL8A2* gene may be involved.[6] Examination of family pedigrees supports a classic autosomal dominant pattern.[7–10] A mitochondrial cause for Fuchs dystrophy has also been reported.[11]

4-2-2 Histopathology

The primary site of disease in Fuchs dystrophy is the endothelial cell. The dystrophy is characterized by a slow continuous loss of morphologically and physiologically altered endothelial cells, eventually leading to corneal edema. The endothelial cells synthesize a thickened Descemet's membrane, with focal excrescences of altered basement membrane material (Figure 4-1).[12]

By light microscopy, endothelial cells exhibit polymegathism, as well as pleomorphism, since they are stretched and their nuclei are pushed into the valleys between developing guttae. By scanning electron microscopy, these outpouchings are better demonstrated (Figure 4-2). There is generalized cellular thinning over the apices of the guttate excrescences (Figure 4-3), with an overall reduction in the endothelial cell count.

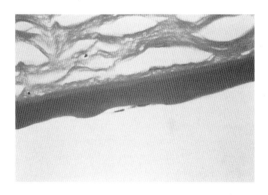

Figure 4-3 *Fuchs endothelial dystrophy. Light microscopy showing excrescences.*

Borderie et al suggested that apoptosis plays a notable role in the degeneration of corneal endothelial cells in Fuchs dystrophy.[13] Some of the endothelial cells take on morphologic features of fibroblasts and produce collagen.[14] Descemet's membrane becomes diffusely thickened because of the deposition of collagenous basement membrane–like material on the posterior surface. In Fuchs dystrophy, the 100- to 110-nm anterior banded portion of Descemet's membrane is entirely normal. The posterior nonbanded layer, however, is thinned or absent and replaced by a posterior banded layer.[15,16]

The anterior banded layer of Descemet's membrane is secreted from the fourth fetal month until close to term. At the time of birth, the endothelial cells switch to synthesis of a homogeneous amorphous type IV basement membrane collagen. This will compose the posterior nonbanded layer of Descemet's membrane. Unlike the anterior banded layer, the posterior nonbanded layer increases slowly throughout life. The width of the two layers can be used to date approximately when synthesis of abnormal Descemet's membrane began.[17] Thus, the thinness of the posterior nonbanded layer in Fuchs dystrophy suggests that endothelial cell function becomes abnormal at an early age (even as early as age 20). Several studies found no evidence of alterations in aqueous humor composition, supporting the notion that Fuchs dystrophy is a primary disorder of the corneal endothelium.[18]

4-2-3 Clinical Manifestations

The initial presentation of Fuchs dystrophy is central corneal guttae. These guttae can be seen as dark spots on the posterior corneal surface by direct illumination on slit-lamp examination. On retroillumination, they resemble dewdrops (Figure 4-4). Often, pigment dusting can be present on the endothelium and may be seen with or without associated corneal guttae. If the guttae coalesce, a classic beaten-metal appearance (due to the increased pigmentation) of the endothelium can be appreciated. Eventually, Descemet's membrane becomes visibly thickened. At this stage of the disease, the first stage, the patient is asymptomatic, but manifests central irregularly distributed guttate warts (Figure 4-5).

Once endothelial cell function is sufficiently compromised, the patient develops stromal and epithelial edema, with symptoms of glare and hazy vision. Visual acuity is reduced at this stage. As the corneal edema increases, the stroma thickens centrally and the edema spreads peripherally. As the stromal edema increases, Descemet's membrane develops folds and vision falls. With time, the epithelium becomes involved and microcystic epithelial edema ensues (Figure 4-6). Topical fluorescein can be helpful in demonstrating this bedewing, by producing dark gaps in the fluorescein film (negative fluorescein staining). Eventually, bullous keratopathy results and these bullae can rupture.

At first, epithelial edema occurs only in the morning, clearing as the day progresses. This happens because the tear film becomes hypotonic due to the lack of evaporation associated with eyelid closure during sleep, thereby preventing water loss from the

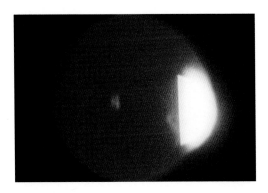

Figure 4-4 *Fuchs endothelial dystrophy. Retroillumination showing guttae.*

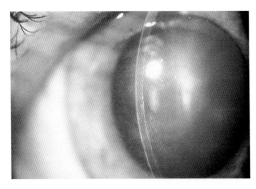

Figure 4-5 *Fuchs endothelial dystrophy. Guttae in early stage of disease.*

corneal epithelium. Environmental factors such as extremes in temperate climates can also affect vision (for example, high humidity). Eventually, the benefit of better vision late in the day is lost, the epithelium becomes more bullous, and pain and photophobia develop.

Stromal edema is more likely to occur with decreased endothelial cell density, but the density is variable. The number of corneal guttae, however, does not appear to correlate well; that is, stromal edema can occur even in the absence of guttae.[19]

In a study by Oh et al, the association between corneal thickness and epithelial edema was assessed using ultrasound pachymetry.[20] The mean corneal thickness was significantly higher (P = 0.002) in the edematous group (mean = 0.682 mm) than in the group without epithelial edema (mean = 0.624 mm). Corneal thickness greater than 0.650 mm was associated with the greatest probability (85%) of corneal edema. Corneal guttae diameter was also assessed for correlation with corneal thickness, but diameter was not significantly cor-

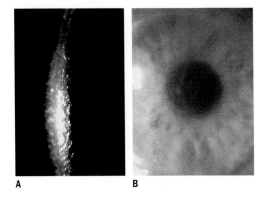

A   B

Figure 4-6 *Fuchs endothelial dystrophy. Microcystic epithelial corneal edema in later stage of disease. (A) Slit-lamp view of microcystic edema. (B) Diffuse illumination demonstrating microcystic edema.*

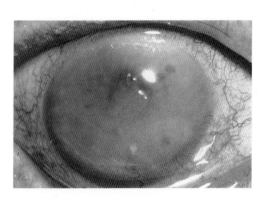

Figure 4-7 *Fuchs endothelial dystrophy. Dense gray sheet of corneal scar tissue in end stage of disease.*

related with thickness ($P = 0.269$). Indeed, there is a demonstrable association between epithelial edema and the measured thickness of the cornea; the corneal guttae diameter itself does not correlate with corneal thickness.

In end-stage Fuchs dystrophy, subepithelial fibrous scarring appears centrally. This is an avascular tissue that does not migrate from the periphery like pannus, but arises in the central cornea. Clinically, it appears as an irregular dense gray sheet of scar tissue (Figure 4-7). Histologically, it consists of active fibroblasts between the epithelium and Bowman's layer.

Subepithelial scarring generally eliminates the recurrent erosions; the stromal edema and epithelial bullae disappear as the stroma scars. The patient becomes more comfortable, but the surface irregularity and loss of corneal transparency further reduce vision. The association of Fuchs dystrophy with glaucoma has been disputed and not established.[21–25]

The progression of Fuchs dystrophy from asymptomatic stage I disease to end-stage disease with subepithelial fibrosis can span an interval of 10 to 20 years. Fortunately, due to the improved success of corneal transplantation, end-stage Fuchs dystrophy is infrequently seen today (Table 4-1 and Figure 4-8).

4-2-4 Management

Fuchs endothelial dystrophy is a significant cause of corneal blindness in the United States. The frequency of corneal guttae in patients over 40 years of age has been reported to be as low as 10%[26] and as high as 70%,[27] depending on the clinical definition of guttae. There are no clinical characteristics of corneal guttae that allow the prediction of corneal edema.

The treatment for Fuchs endothelial dystrophy varies, depending on the severity of the disease. The medical management of Fuchs dystrophy with visually significant corneal edema includes the use of topical hyperosmotic agents (for example, topical sodium chloride 5%), corneal dehydration with a blow-dryer at arm's length, as well as reduction of IOP. NaCl 5% drops are prescribed 4 to 8 times per day, with NaCl 5% ointment at bedtime. A hair dryer, held at arm's length, helps dry out the corneal surface. Lowering IOP appears to have limited usefulness. Although topical corticosteroids are generally believed to have no role in Fuchs dystrophy, they may have a limited role in the treatment of early Fuchs dystrophy by increasing Na$^+$/K$^+$-ATPase pump site density.[28,29]

Other forms of medical management include the use of a therapeutic bandage contact lens to alleviate discomfort resulting from recurrent erosions caused by epithelial bullae and rupture. This temporary form of treatment is particularly beneficial in making patients awaiting corneal transplantation more comfortable.

Despite the different methods of medical management for Fuchs dystrophy, penetrating keratoplasty is the treatment of choice for patients with reduction in vision sufficient to impair activities of daily living. Fuchs dystrophy is the third most common indication, after pseudophakic bullous keratopathy and failed graft, for penetrating keratoplasty.[30,31] Fuchs dystrophy accounts for about 5.8% to 15% of all penetrating keratoplasties performed in the United States.[32–36] The reported percentage appears to be fairly constant across Western

TABLE 4-1

Clinical Staging of Fuchs Endothelial Dystrophy

Stage	Vision	Symptoms	Slit Lamp
1	Unaffected	Asymptomatic	Central guttae Thickened Descemet's membrane
2	Decreased, worse in morning	Glare with or without pain, worse in morning	Stromal edema Microcysts Bullae
3	Poor	No pain	Subepithelial fibrosis

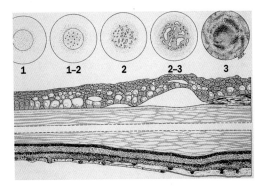

Figure 4-8 *Fuchs endothelial dystrophy. Timeline of events corresponding to clinical stages in Table 4-1.*

societies: 13.9% in Denmark,[35] 8.0% in
Scotland,[37] and 8.3% in France.[38] Other surgical treatment options, short of penetrating keratoplasty, include microkeratome-
assisted posterior lamellar keratoplasty,
amniotic membrane graft for persistent
keratoepithelial defect, conjunctival flap,
anterior stromal puncture, or phototherapeutic keratectomy for anterior stromal
scarring.

The prognosis for surgery in Fuchs dystrophy is good, with clear grafts reported in
80% to 90% of patients at 5 years and a
somewhat lower percentage long-term.[39–42]
The results of penetrating keratoplasty for
Fuchs dystrophy compare favorably with
the results of other common indications for
the procedure, such as pseudophakic bullous keratopathy and herpetic keratopathy.

The decision whether to perform combined corneal transplantation and cataract
extraction with intraocular lens implanta-
tion (triple procedure) can be a difficult
one. Two clinical situations arise that con-
front the clinician with this dilemma. In
one instance, the patient with a visually significant cataract has borderline endothelial
function. The second is the patient with
corneal edema who has a mild-to-moderate
cataract.

The majority of patients with confluent
guttae who exhibit no evidence of stromal
edema tend to do well with cataract surgery
alone. These patients should, however, be
counseled on the risk of corneal decompensation following cataract extraction. In a retrospective chart review of 236 patients with
Fuchs dystrophy and cataracts, Pineros et al
found no statistically significant difference
in the outcome and refractive status after
triple versus nonsimultaneous procedures.[43]
To avoid increased cost and delay in visual
rehabilitation, the authors recommend a
triple procedure for patients with Fuchs
endothelial dystrophy and visually significant cataracts.

In the case of corneal edema without visually significant cataract, the surgeon must
weigh the added intraoperative risk of
cataract extraction, as well as the unpre-
dictability of postoperative refractive error
in a triple procedure. Payant et al performed a retrospective analysis of 78 eyes in
58 patients who underwent corneal transplantation for Fuchs endothelial dystrophy
without cataract extraction.[44] These patients were examined for the presence of
cataract after corneal transplantation. Followup ranged from 1 to 17 years, with an
average of 6.62 years. Of the 78 eyes, 44%
developed cataracts sufficient enough to require surgical removal. The mean time
from transplant to cataract formation aver-
aged 4.9 years. Age and length of followup
were statistically significant risk factors.
The incidence of cataract after penetrating
keratoplasty increased at age 50 and occurred in 75% of eyes grafted after 60 years
of age. If followup was long enough, more
than 90% of patients developed a cataract
at 15 years.

CONGENITAL HEREDITARY ENDOTHELIAL DYSTROPHY

4-3-1 Genetics and Causation

Congenital hereditary endothelial dystrophy (CHED) is an inherited bilateral congenital, relatively nonprogressive, symmetric corneal edema resulting from a primary endothelial dysfunction. CHED is characterized by corneal opacification that ranges from a diffuse haze to a ground-glass milky appearance. CHED is rare in most countries, but is the second most frequent corneal dystrophy in Saudi Arabia, mostly the result of consanguineous marriages.[45]

Judisch and Maumenee recognized both autosomal dominant and autosomal recessive types of CHED.[46] They reviewed a series of published reports in which familial cases revealed that corneal clouding in autosomal recessive CHED was present at birth or in the neonatal period. Furthermore, corneal changes with time were minimal, nystagmus was often present, and there were no other signs or symptoms. On the other hand, in autosomal dominant CHED, the cornea was clear at birth, corneal opacification was slowly progressive, and nystagmus was mostly absent. As the authors noted, usually little or no congenital evidence exists for the dominant type. They proposed that "infantile" or "autosomal dominant" CHED would be a more appropriate term for the dominant variant.

The genes responsible for both autosomal dominant (AD) CHED and autosomal recessive (AR) CHED have now been identified. AD-CHED (CHED1) has been mapped to the pericentromeric region of chromosome 20. Hand et al investigated a large, consanguineous Irish pedigree with AR-CHED, excluding linkage to the AD-CHED locus.[47] Evidence for linkage to chromosome 20p was demonstrated. This AR-CHED (CHED2) disease gene locus is physically and genetically distinct from the AD-CHED locus. Indeed, CHED1 (AD) has been mapped to the pericentromeric region of chromosome 20 (20p11.2-q11.2) in an area overlapping a gene for autosomal dominant posterior polymorphous dystrophy (PPMD). The gene for CHED2 (AR) is located in the telomeric portion of chromosome 20.[48,49] Conventional genetic analysis, in addition to a pooled DNA strategy, excluded linkage of AR-CHED to the AD-CHED and larger PPMD loci. This demonstrates that AR-CHED is genetically distinct from AD-CHED and PPMD.[48]

Kanis et al sought to determine whether AR-CHED segregating in a consanguineous Saudi Arabian pedigree was linked to the previously mapped and overlapping loci for AD-CHED and PPMD on the pericentromeric region of chromosome 20.[50] Analysis of the genotype data with the MENDEL software package, utilizing a model of autosomal recessive inheritance with complete penetrance, showed exclusion of CHED from PPMD/AD-CHED. Their results showed that AR-CHED is not allelic to either AD-CHED or PPMD, although it has been proposed that AD-CHED may be allelic to PPMD. Thus, there are at least two distinct genes responsible for CHED and PPMD.

4-3-2 Histopathology

The essential feature of CHED is bilateral diffuse corneal edema unrelated to commonly known causative factors (for example, congenital glaucoma or intrauterine infection). This condition results from degeneration of the endothelium, which may occur in utero or within the first year of life. Endothelial cells are either atrophic or completely absent.

Patients with CHED have a markedly increased corneal thickness (0.93 to 0.98 mm), with epithelial edema and a stromal swelling pressure close to zero, suggesting that the stroma is maximally swollen in vivo. Indeed, the most characteristic feature of CHED is stromal thickening, with severe disorganization and disruption of the lamellar pattern. The corneal endothelium shows an increased permeability to fluorescein, thus suggesting a functional barrier defect.[51]

The endothelium in most reported cases of CHED either has been absent or has had a greatly reduced number of cells. In one study, the endothelial cells did not grow even when placed in tissue culture media.[52]

In a study by Ehlers et al, histopathologic evaluation in CHED revealed the following[51]:

1. Normal endothelial cell density

2. Abnormal endothelial morphology, with irregular and multinucleated cells containing abnormal cell organelles

3. Profound thickening of Descemet's membrane, 16 to 18 μm, with multiple focal areas of abnormal fibrillar deposits in the posterior half of the membrane

These findings suggest that the primary defect in CHED is a degenerated and dysfunctional corneal endothelium, characterized by increased permeability and abnormal and accelerated Descemet's membrane secretion. Other investigators have confirmed similar findings: that the endothelial cells in CHED are functionally and morphologically abnormal.[52–55] The defective endothelium fails to produce a normal Descemet's membrane and cannot maintain the cornea in a nonedematous state.

The posterior collagenous layer of Descemet's membrane contains collagen types I, III–V, as well as laminin. The distribution of collagen types I, III, and V within the posterior collagenous layer of Descemet's membrane supports morphologic observations of fibroblast-like changes of the endothelium in CHED.[56]

The anterior 100- to 110-nm banded portion of Descemet's membrane is normal, indicating that endothelial function is preserved, at least through the fifth month of gestation. After that time, a defective endothelium secretes abnormal and excessive basement membrane. The nonbanded posterior portions of Descemet's membrane accumulate this aberrant, abnormal, and excessive basement membrane.[52,57,58] These endothelial abnormalities in CHED become manifest in utero after the fetal anterior portion of Descemet's membrane is synthesized.

4-3-3 Clinical Manifestations

CHED reportedly can be inherited in both autosomal dominant and autosomal recessive forms. The autosomal dominant type (CHED1) is slowly progressive and presents during the first 2 years of life with photophobia and tearing. Autosomal recessive CHED (CHED2) becomes evident at, or shortly after, birth and does not appear to show a progressive course. Nystagmus is absent in CHED1, but is a feature of CHED2.[49] The recessive form of CHED is more common and more severe. Bilateral corneal clouding can range from a mild haze to a milky ground-glass opacification (Figure 4-9).

CHED is a diagnosis of exclusion; other causes of congenital corneal clouding must be ruled out first: congenital glaucoma, forceps injury, congenital infections, early-onset PPMD, and metabolic diseases. Generally, no other anterior or posterior segment abnormalities are associated.

Differentiation of CHED from congenital glaucoma should not be difficult because of the increased IOP in glaucoma, as well as the increased corneal diameter. In CHED, the corneal diameter is not enlarged and the IOP is normal. There are, however, reported cases of the two conditions occurring together.[59,60]

Pedersen et al described a patient with congenital glaucoma and iris hypoplasia who underwent repeated surgery to control the glaucoma and whose corneas progressively opacified; the patient subsequently underwent bilateral penetrating keratoplasty.[59] Histopathologic studies demon-

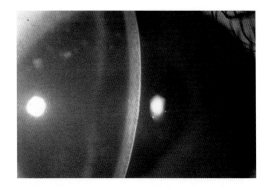

Figure 4-9 *Congenital hereditary endothelial dystrophy. Diffuse corneal edema.*
Courtesy Richard K. Forster, MD, from King Khaled Eye Specialist Hospital, Riyadh, Saudi Arabia.

strated specific changes of Descemet's membrane and the endothelium that were typical of CHED. Mullaney et al described 3 patients with a clear association between congenital glaucoma and CHED.[60] The combination should be suspected where persistent and total corneal opacification fails to resolve after normalization of IOP.

Asymptomatic relatives of patients with CHED can manifest corneal changes resembling those of PPMD.[61] According to a study by Levenson et al, the offspring of these individuals appear to be at a higher risk for developing CHED.[62]

4-3-4 Management

The only available treatment for CHED is penetrating keratoplasty. Most early reports suggest a poor prognosis for corneal transplantation in CHED.[61,63] In the series by Pearce et al, only 9 of 21 grafts remained clear for more than 3 months.[61] In later cases, the outcomes after penetrating keratoplasty were much more favorable[64,65] and the percentage of grafts that survived to 5 years was about 60% to 70%.[65,66] Surgical success was better in cases of delayed onset compared with early congenital onset. Early surgical intervention was recommended to prevent the development or progression of amblyopia.[65–67]

POSTERIOR POLYMORPHOUS DYSTROPHY

4-4-1 Genetics and Causation

Posterior polymorphous dystrophy (PPMD) is a bilateral autosomal dominantly inherited posterior membrane dystrophy. It is clinically recognized by the presence of vesicles on the endothelial surface of the cornea. The corneal endothelium is normally a single layer of cells, which lose their mitotic potential after development is complete. In PPMD, the endothelium is often multilayered and has several other characteristics of an epithelium, including the presence of desmosomes, tonofilaments, and microvilli.[68] The cells lining the posterior surface of the cornea have a varied appearance clinically, and the corneal endothelial cells possess features of epithelial cells (epithelialization of the endothelium). These abnormal endothelial cells retain their ability to divide and can extend onto the trabecular meshwork, resulting in glaucoma in up to 40% of cases.

PPMD was first described by Koeppe in 1916 under the name *keratitis bullosa interna*.[69] In 1969, Pearce et al reported a family in which 39 persons in 5 generations were affected.[61] The investigators noted an unequal sex ratio in the offspring of affected females: more females were affected, with a paucity of affected males. No biologic explanation could be found, and it was concluded that this unequal sex ratio was a chance occurrence. They termed the condition *congenital endothelial corneal dystrophy*.

Héon et al studied a large family with 21 members affected with PPMD.[70] This family was genotyped using short-tandem repeat polymorphisms distributed across the autosomal genome. Linkage was established with markers on the long arm of chromosome 20. The gene responsible for PPMD has now been mapped to the pericentromeric region of human chromosome 20 (20q11).[47,49] Blood relatives of affected persons may have CHED1, suggesting that the two disorders may be related. This possibility is supported by the mapping of a CHED1 gene to the same region of chromosome 20.[49]

4-4-2 Histopathology

Since PPMD is usually asymptomatic, corneal tissue has been examined only in cases severe enough to require penetrating keratoplasty.[71] As indicated by the word *polymorphous*, PPMD is characterized by deep corneal lesions of various shapes. Nodular grouped vesicular and blister-like lesions commonly occur. The posterior surface of the cornea tends to be covered by a geographic pattern of endothelial and epithelial-like cells, sometimes creating vesicles and sometimes creating partly detached sheets of cells.[72] An irregularly thickened multilaminar Descemet's membrane occasionally contains focal nodular excrescences (similar to guttae), but true corneal guttae are absent. The corneal epithelium and stroma show no remarkable features in PPMD, with the exception of chronic edema in more severe cases.

Electron microscopic studies have revealed the main abnormality to be within the endothelial cell.[72–74] Boruchoff and Kuwabara showed that, in focal areas, the endothelium in PPMD contains large squamous epithelial cells.[75] These islands of epithelium-like endothelial cells (Figure 4-10) tend to be multilayered, with extensive microvilli, desmosomal junctions, and

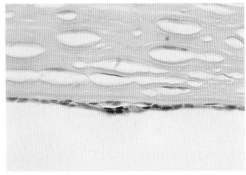

A

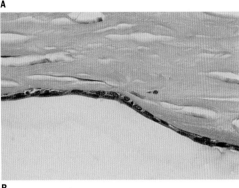

B

Figure 4-10 *Posterior polymorphous dystrophy. Light microscopy showing (A) multilayered epithelialized endothelial cells and (B) epithelialization of endothelium.*

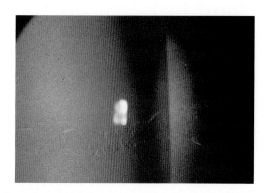

Figure 4-11 *Posterior polymorphous dystrophy. Retro-illumination showing band-like structures.*

tonofilaments. The presence of unusual epithelial-like endothelial cells has been confirmed by several reports using both transmission and scanning electron microscopy.[73,76,77]

Band-like structures clinically similar to Haab's striae occur in PPMD (Figure 4-11) and can result in confusion of the two entities. The difference in clinical appearance is based on differences in histopathology. The edges of Haab's striae are thickened and curled, and they secondarily proliferate Descemet's membrane. The area between the edges is thin and smooth. In PPMD, the exact opposite occurs: the band is a thickening of Descemet's membrane between the edges, with thinner and more normal Descemet's membrane outside the band.[78] These endothelial bands (gray lines) in Descemet's membrane have the appearance of railroad tracks.

Descemet's membrane in most cases of PPMD has the normal 100- to 110-nm anterior banded zone,[68,79] as is normal for this zone throughout life. Since the anterior banded zone of Descemet's membrane is secreted between the third or fourth month of fetal life and term, a normal anterior banded zone is strong evidence that the endothelial cells were functionally normal prenatally.[80] The abnormality in PPMD most likely develops late in gestation or shortly after birth.

4-4-3 Clinical Manifestations

As stated earlier, PPMD is transmitted in an autosomal dominant fashion. The dystrophy usually manifests bilaterally, but asymmetric unilateral presentation has been documented.[75] Most patients with PPMD, however, are asymptomatic and

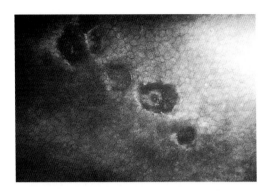

Figure 4-12 *Posterior polymorphous dystrophy. Specular microscopy showing vesicular lesions.*

have normal vision. PPMD tends to be nonprogressive or very slowly progressive.

Deep corneal lesions of various shapes characterize PPMD, including nodular, vesicular, and blister-like lesions (Figure 4-12). The hallmark of PPMD is the vesicular lesion, which does not necessarily occur in all patients. These vesicles can be found throughout the posterior cornea and can be isolated, in clusters, or confluent.[68,79,81,82] The spectrum of clinical presentations in PPMD is shown in Figure 4-13.

Slit-lamp findings include corneal edema in more advanced cases, calcific and stromal lipid degenerative changes in severe cases, band-like lesions at the level of Descemet's membrane lined by pleomorphic endothelial cells, localized or diffuse thickening of Descemet's membrane, classic posterior corneal vesicular lesions, and islands of abnormal cells surrounded by normal-appearing endothelial cells. The severity of the iridocorneal adhesions ranges from fine or broad-based adhesions seen only on gonioscopy to large iridocorneal adhesions seen easily by slit-lamp examination. All

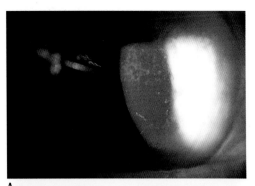

A

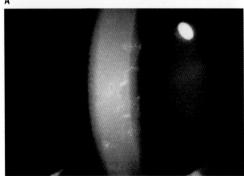

B

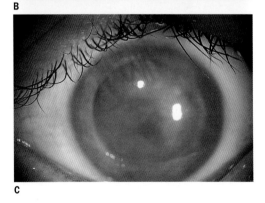

C

Figure 4-13 *Posterior polymorphous dystrophy. Spectrum of clinical presentations. (A) Posterior "train-track" linear lines and vesicles. (B) Mild corneal edema. (C) Significant endothelial and stromal opacity at late stage.*

patients with broad-based iridocorneal adhesions have elevated IOP.[68]

Elevated IOP occurs in about 15% of cases.[68,75,81,83,84] This association can occur either with anatomically open angles or with angle closure. The mechanism for angle closure can be easily understood, as it is due to endothelial migration across the trabecular meshwork, resulting in peripheral anterior synechial closure.[85,86] Open-angle glaucoma has been suggested to result from high iris insertion, resulting in compression to the trabecular meshwork.[87]

In addition to the association with glaucoma, PPMD has been associated with anterior segment dysgenesis, including abnormal iris processes, iris atrophy, pupillary ectropion, glass-like membranes on the anterior iris surface, and bands in Descemet's membrane.[81,88,89] Other disorders that have been reported in association with PPMD include band keratopathy,[89] calcium deposition of the deep stroma,[90] posterior keratoconus,[91–93] posterior amyloid degeneration,[94] Terrien marginal degeneration,[95] and Alport syndrome.[96]

As with CHED, PPMD must be differentiated from other congenital disorders that result in a cloudy cornea at birth, including CHED, congenital glaucoma, sclerocornea, congenital infection, and metabolic disease. In addition, PPMD must be differentiated from iridocorneal endothelial (ICE) syndrome, with which it shares many clinical features.

Features that PPMD and ICE share include iridocorneal adhesions, iris atrophy, corectopia, ectropion uveae, elevated IOP, and corneal edema. PPMD by definition is a dystrophy, indicating familial inheritance and bilateral occurrence. ICE syndrome, on the other hand, is generally a unilateral sporadic occurrence. However, this distinction can become less clear when ICE syndrome manifests bilaterally.[97–101] For patients in whom the clinical distinction cannot be made with certainty, specular microscopy can help differentiate ICE from PPMD.[82,102]

4-4-4 Management

The overwhelming majority of patients with PPMD remain asymptomatic and stable. In a small number of patients, however, this dystrophy can be visually significant, extensive, and progressive, thus necessitating surgical intervention. In the largest series of PPMD cases reported, only 13 of 120 individuals required penetrating keratoplasty.[68] The clinically significant corneal edema that develops in this small number of patients generally necessitates a corneal graft by middle age. Early manifestation of PPMD, with corneal edema presenting at birth or soon after, is extremely rare: only a few ultrastructural reports are available.[103]

The prognosis for surgery is strongly correlated with the presence of peripheral anterior synechiae, as well as elevated IOP. In a study by Krachmer, visible retrocorneal membranes formed in 4 of the 22 grafts performed on patients with PPMD.[68] All 4 of these eyes had preoperative iridocorneal adhesions visible on slit-lamp examination; 3 of the 4 grafts failed. In addition, of the 9

TABLE 4-2

Comparison of Endothelial Corneal Dystrophies (AD = autosomal dominant.
AR = autosomal recessive.)

Characteristic	Fuchs Endothelial Dystrophy	Congenital Hereditary Endothelial Dystrophy	Posterior Polymorphous Dystrophy
Inheritance	AD	AD AR	AD
Gene locus	1p34.3-p32 20	20p (type I) 20 tel (type II)	20q11
Onset	Fifth decade	From birth to first year	Second decade Rarely at birth
Progression	Variable	Minimal	Slow or nonprogressive
Corneal thickness	Increased	Increased	Normal
Location	Central	Diffuse	Diffuse
Corneal appearance	Endothelial excrescences	Ground-glass appearance	Vesicles Ground-glass appearance Bands ("railroad tracks") With or without peripheral anterior synechiae
Histology	Guttae Compromised endothelial function with low endothelial cell density	Absent or markedly abnormal endothelium	Abnormal, atrophic endothelium (epithelialization of endothelium)
Surgical prognosis	Very good, but long-term more guarded	Fair to good Guarded in pediatric age group	Good if no peripheral anterior synechiae or elevated IOP

grafts (41%) that failed, glaucoma was involved in 6 of the 9 (27% of all 22 grafts). It appears the factor that most prominently influences the prognosis for penetrating keratoplasty is the preoperative presence of iridocorneal adhesions, as well as elevated IOP.

Table 4-2 summarizes the differences among the endothelial dystrophies.

IRIDOCORNEAL ENDOTHELIAL SYNDROME

4-5-1 Genetics and Causation

Although iridocorneal endothelial (ICE) syndrome is not a true endothelial dystrophy, its chief characteristics—endothelial abnormalities, peripheral anterior synechiae, glaucoma, iris atrophy, and iris nodules—place this entity in the same differential diagnosis as the endothelial dystrophies. ICE syndrome is a nonfamilial unilateral disorder that is more common in women and is usually diagnosed between 30 and 50 years of age. It consists of three different clinical entities:

1. Chandler syndrome
2. Essential (progressive) iris atrophy
3. Cogan-Reese (iris nevus) syndrome

These three clinical conditions are commonly grouped together into a single syndrome because they have similar pathologic processes.[104–106] Langova et al believe that essential iris atrophy, Chandler syndrome, and iris nevus syndrome represent a spectrum of pathologic processes that include a corneal endothelial proliferation with dramatic iris changes.[107] They prefer the term *primary proliferative endothelial degeneration*, which emphasizes the pathogenic origin of the corneal endothelial proliferation.

In essential iris atrophy, iris features predominate: iris atrophy, iris hole formation, and corectopia.[108] In Chandler syndrome, corneal endothelial changes predominate and iris features are mild or absent.[109] In the iris nevus syndrome, nodular pigmented elevations are present on the iris and corneal changes may or may not be present.[110]

Ischemic, toxic, and inflammatory causes have been considered and dismissed.[106] Several reports have proposed and supported a viral causation. Using the polymerase chain reaction, Alvarado et al confirmed the presence of herpes simplex virus (HSV) DNA in the endothelium of a large percentage of ICE syndrome patients.[111] Their results provide direct evidence to support the hypothesis that ICE syndrome has a viral origin. Other investigators have supported these findings. Groh et al detected the presence of HSV in the aqueous humor of patients with ICE syndrome.[112] Although both groups of investigators have data to support evidence of HSV DNA in ICE syndrome, these findings have not been invariably present.

Since the corneal endothelium is derived from neural crest cells, endothelial metaplastic transformation has received considerable attention.[98,113–115] Howell et al believe that the epithelial-like endothelial cells in ICE syndrome are cells of endothelial lineage, rather than a heterotopia of epithelial cells.[113] Their data support the hypothesis that the abnormal cells in ICE syndrome arise by way of a metaplastic transformation of pre-existing endothelium.

Strong evidence exists to indicate that ICE syndrome is nonfamilial[82,116,117] and unilateral.[102,116,117] There are, however, many case reports in the literature of familial or bilateral involvement.[97–101,118–120] Although the exact cause of ICE syndrome has not been confirmed, it is believed that some event incites the endothelium and basement membrane to extend beyond the peripheral cornea, leading to the formation of peripheral anterior synechiae and glaucoma. Whether the inciting event is viral in origin, a metaplastic transformation of neural crest cells, a combination of the two, or some other process has yet to be confirmed.

4-5-2 Histopathology

The primary abnormality in ICE syndrome is a defect in the corneal endothelium.[102] The abnormal endothelial cells can be present on the trabecular meshwork, the anterior surface of the iris, and the posterior corneal surface.[105,106,114,121,122] These corneal endothelial cells are diminished in number, irregular in shape, and demonstrate epithelial features: microvilli, cytoplasmic tonofilaments, and desmosomal junctions.[114,121,123] Ultrastructural changes in the endothelial cells, as well as abnormalities observed in Descemet's membrane, suggest that the endothelial cells are normal initially, but subsequently acquire epithelial-like features.[124] With confocal microscopy, the characteristic epithelioid changes of the endothelium can be demonstrated.[125] Descemet's membrane may be normal or thickened, but it contains an abnormal posterior collagenous layer. This extracellular matrix is composed of wide-spaced type VIII collagen.[126,127]

Hirst et al demonstrated an almost universal staining of the corneal endothelial layer with AE1 and AE3 keratin monoclonal antibodies, as well as vimentin.[114] Endothelial features consistent with keratin were confirmed through the use of transmission electron microscopy (TEM). The endothelial cell layer in ICE syndrome has electron microscopic and immunohistochemical characteristics of epithelial-like cells, but its cross-reactivity with vimentin suggests that these cells retain (or derive) some endothelial staining characteristics.

Using immunocytochemical studies, other investigators have demonstrated similar findings. Levy et al showed that cells in ICE syndrome were morphologically similar to epithelial cells and expressed the same profile of differentiation markers as normal limbal epithelial cells.[128] Other histopathologic studies performed by Levy et al have demonstrated a population of well-differentiated cells with epithelial features: desmosomes, tonofilaments, and microvilli.[129] Despite having epithelial features, these epithelial-like endothelial cells are of endothelial lineage.[113]

4-5-3 Clinical Manifestations

ICE syndrome is characterized clinically by a hammered-silver appearance of the corneal endothelium, corneal failure, glaucoma, and iris destruction.[129] The most common corneal abnormality is a fine hammered-metal appearance of the endothelium.[129,130] Stromal or epithelial edema, peripheral anterior synechiae, endothelial abnormalities, and even superficial band keratopathy may develop (Figure 4-14). Generally, there is diffuse involvement of the corneal endothelium, but focal areas of involvement have been described.[117,125]

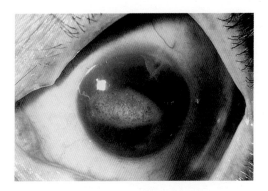

Figure 4-14 *Iridocorneal endothelial syndrome. Clinical appearance of cornea, with chronic corneal edema, iris atrophy, endothelial abnormalities, peripheral anterior synechiae, and band keratopathy.*

The diagnosis of ICE syndrome is made when two of three main clinical features are present: corneal endothelial abnormalities, iris changes, and peripheral anterior synechiae.[106,116,130,131] Correctly identifying a particular subtype is not necessary, since management is geared toward the dominant clinical features.

ICE syndrome is a progressive disorder, but the subtypes of the syndrome may be variable in progression. Careful slit-lamp examination and gonioscopy, with clear chart documentation at regular intervals, are indispensable for the assessment of progression.

More severe cases are characterized by peripheral anterior synechiae formation, progressive atrophy of the iris stroma, and stretching of the iris (Figure 4-15). The synechiae are usually visible without gonioscopy but, as mentioned, gonioscopic examination forms an integral part of the ophthalmologic examination in patients with ICE syndrome. Pupil eccentricity is found in the direction of the most prominent synechiae. Elevated IOP is common, and glaucoma may be an early or late finding (depending on the degree of trabecular meshwork involvement and synechiae formation), often requiring surgical intervention.

4-5-4 Management

Depending on the extent of the disease, corneal edema and secondary glaucoma are both treated primarily by medical or surgical reduction of IOP. Penetrating keratoplasty is occasionally required for patients with advanced corneal edema.[106] Treatment is geared toward the dominant clinical features.

Until further studies corroborate the role of a specific viral causation (for example, HSV), antiviral therapy cannot be advocated.[111] Medical treatment is of limited value. Fulcher et al have data to suggest that an immunotoxin (454A12-rRTA)—antitransferrin receptor monoclonal antibody (454A12) conjugated to recombinant ricin A chain (rRTA)—may be used to inhibit growth of proliferating human corneal endothelium in pathologic conditions such as ICE syndrome.[132] Further research in this area is required before immunomodulating factors can be recommended.

Control of IOP can occasionally be achieved medically. Given the pathophysiology of ICE syndrome, it should be no surprise that the most effective antiglaucoma agents are the aqueous suppressants. Since the problem is one of access to the trabecular meshwork, pilocarpine and miotics are ineffective. The role of aqueous suppressants is generally short-lived (due to progressive angle closure). Laser trabeculoplasty is generally not effective.[133] Glaucoma filtering surgery (trabeculectomy), however, does offer a reasonable chance for success.

Patients with ICE syndrome are at higher risk for failure with glaucoma filtering procedures.[134] In addition to the usual causes of bleb failure, endothelialization of the bleb has been reported to be a source of bleb failure.[105,135–137] The success rates for subsequent surgeries are comparable to those of initial surgery in patients with primary open-angle glaucoma.[137] Given the higher risk for bleb failure, some authors have advocated trabeculectomy with mitomycin C application. The addition of an antimetabolite seems to offer a reasonable

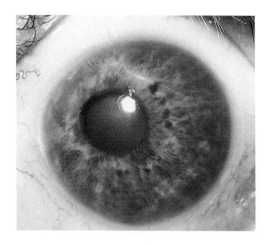

Figure 4-15 *Iridocorneal endothelial syndrome. Iris stretching.*

intermediate-term success rate for ICE syndrome patients.[138] Another option, aqueous shunt surgery, appears to be an effective method for IOP lowering in some eyes with ICE syndrome–related glaucoma when medical treatment or conventional filtration surgeries fail. Additional glaucoma procedures and/or aqueous shunt revisions with tube repositionings should be anticipated.[139]

Lowering IOP can reduce corneal edema. Despite IOP reduction, penetrating keratoplasty is often required. It is an effective treatment of corneal endothelial decompensation in ICE syndrome.[140] The prognosis for penetrating keratoplasty in this syndrome appears to be very favorable in the majority of eyes.[116,131,141] In a retrospective chart review of 9 patients with ICE syndrome, Crawford et al observed that penetrating keratoplasty resulted in visual improvement in 7 of the 9, with relief of pain in all 6 of the patients who had pain (mean followup was 43 months).[116]

The prognosis for the procedure in essential iris atrophy, however, appears to be more guarded, in that penetrating keratoplasty is frequently associated with chronic anterior uveitis and immunologic graft failure.[142] Penetrating keratoplasty is a relatively safe and effective procedure for patients with diminished vision or other complaints related to corneal abnormalities in ICE syndrome. It does not, however, restore to normal the iris and angle structures affected adversely by the progression of the corneal endotheliopathy. Other measures may be required to control IOP.[141] The two major factors attributed to poor visual acuity after surgery include glaucoma and graft failure (immune and nonimmune). The key determinant in the ultimate visual prognosis of ICE syndrome is adequate control of glaucoma.

4-6

CONCLUSION

Diagnosis and treatment for endothelial corneal dystrophies have improved significantly in the past decade. The mainstay of therapy remains penetrating keratoplasty, although microkeratome-assisted posterior lamellar keratoplasty represents a promising new treatment. The endothelial corneal dystrophies are among the most common clinical indications for penetrating keratoplasty today. With regard to advances in the understanding of molecular causation for this group of diseases, in contrast to anterior corneal dystrophies, limited progress has been made in chromosome linkage and gene identification; much work remains to be done.

REFERENCES

1. Easty DL, Sparrow JM: *Oxford Textbook of Ophthalmology.* New York: Oxford University Press; 1999.

2. Streiff B: [Ernst Fuchs (1851–1930): commemorative lecture, Vienna, 31 May 1984.] *Klin Monatsbl Augenheilkd* 1984;185:316–320.

3. Kruger KE: [In memory of professor Leonhard Koeppe, MD.] *Klin Monatsbl Augenheilkd* 1969;155:147.

4. Schlapfer H, Wagner H: [The 100th anniversary of Prof. Alfred Vogt, 31 October 1879–10 December 1943.] *Schweiz Med Wochenschr* 1979; 109:1565–1566.

5. Hogan MJ, Wood I, Fine M: Fuchs' endothelial dystrophy of the cornea. 29th Sanford Gifford Memorial lecture. *Am J Ophthalmol* 1974;78: 363–383.

6. Biswas S, Munier FL, Yardley J, et al: Missense mutations in COL8A2, the gene encoding the alpha 2 chain of type VIII collagen, cause two forms of corneal endothelial dystrophy. *Hum Mol Genet* 2001;10:2415–2423.

7. Magovern M, Beauchamp GR, McTigue JW, et al: Inheritance of Fuchs' combined dystrophy. *Ophthalmology* 1979;86:1897–1923.

8. Rosenblum P, Stark WJ, Maumenee IH, et al: Hereditary Fuchs' dystrophy. *Am J Ophthalmol* 1980;90:455–462.

9. Krachmer JH, Bucher KD, Purcell JJ Jr, et al: Inheritance of endothelial dystrophy of the cornea. *Ophthalmologica* 1980;181:301–313.

10. Alexandrakis G, Filatov V, Adamis AP: De-novo development of corneal guttae and Fuchs' dystrophy in corneal grafts. *CLAO J* 2000;26: 44–46.

11. Albin RL: Fuchs' corneal dystrophy in a patient with mitochondrial DNA mutations. *J Med Genet* 1998;35:258–259.

12. Adamis AP, Filatov V, Tripathi BJ, et al: Fuchs' endothelial dystrophy of the cornea. *Surv Ophthalmol* 1993;38:149–168.

13. Borderie VM, Baudrimont M, Vallee A, et al: Corneal endothelial cell apoptosis in patients with Fuchs' dystrophy. *Invest Ophthalmol Vis Sci* 2000;41:2501–2505.

14. Iwamoto T, DeVoe AG: Electron microscopic studies on Fuchs' combined dystrophy, I: posterior portion of the cornea. *Invest Ophthalmol* 1971; 10:9–28.

15. Johnson DH, Bourne WM, Campbell RJ: The ultrastructure of Descemet's membrane, I: changes with age in normal corneas. *Arch Ophthalmol* 1982;100:1942–1947.

16. Bourne WM, Johnson DH, Campbell RJ: The ultrastructure of Descemet's membrane, III: Fuchs' dystrophy. *Arch Ophthalmol* 1982;100: 1952–1955.

17. Krachmer JH, Mannis MJ, Holland EJ: *Cornea*. St Louis: CV Mosby Co; 1997.

18. Wilson SE, Bourne WM, Maguire LJ, et al: Aqueous humor composition in Fuchs' dystrophy. *Invest Ophthalmol Vis Sci* 1989;30:449–453.

19. Abbott RL, Fine BS, Webster RG Jr, et al: Specular microscopic and histologic observations in nonguttate corneal endothelial degeneration. *Ophthalmology* 1981;88:788–800.

20. Oh KT, Weil LJ, Oh DM, et al: Corneal thickness in Fuchs' dystrophy with and without epithelial oedema. *Eye* 1998;12:282–284.

21. Buxton JN, Preston RW, Riechers R, et al: Tonography in cornea guttata: a preliminary report. *Arch Ophthalmol* 1967;77:602–603.

22. Roberts CW, Steinert RF, Thomas JV, et al: Endothelial guttata and facility of aqueous outflow. *Cornea* 1984;3:5–9.

23. Krachmer JH, Purcell JJ Jr, Young CW, et al: Corneal endothelial dystrophy: a study of 64 families. *Arch Ophthalmol* 1978;96:2036–2039.

24. Pitts JF, Jay JL: The association of Fuchs' corneal endothelial dystrophy with axial hypermetropia, shallow anterior chamber, and angle closure glaucoma. *Br J Ophthalmol* 1990;74: 601–604.

25. Brooks AM, Grant G, Gillies WE: The significance of anterior chamber depth in Fuchs' corneal dystrophy and cornea guttata. *Cornea* 1994;13:131–135.

26. Goar EL: Dystrophy of the corneal endothelium (corneal guttata), with a report of a histological examination. *Am J Ophthalmol* 1934;17: 215–221.

27. Lorenzetti DW, Votila MH, Parikh N, et al: Central corneal guttata: incidence in the general population. *Am J Ophthalmol* 1967;64:1155–1158.

28. Geroski DH, Matsuda M, Yee RW, et al: Pump function of the human corneal endothelium: effects of age and cornea guttata. *Ophthalmology* 1985;92:759–763.

29. Yee RW, Geroski DH, Matsuda M, et al: Correlation of corneal endothelial pump site density, barrier function, and morphology in wound repair. *Invest Ophthalmol Vis Sci* 1985;26:1191–1201.

30. Patel NP, Kim T, Rapuano CJ, et al: Indications for and outcomes of repeat penetrating keratoplasty, 1989–1995. *Ophthalmology* 2000; 107:719–724.

31. Hyman L, Wittpenn J, Yang C: Indications and techniques of penetrating keratoplasties, 1985–1988. *Cornea* 1992;11:573–576.

32. Robin JB, Gindi JJ, Koh K, et al: An update of the indications for penetrating keratoplasty, 1979 through 1983. *Arch Ophthalmol* 1986;104: 87–89.

33. Mamalis N, Craig MT, Coulter VL, et al: Penetrating keratoplasty, 1981–1988: clinical indications and pathologic findings. *J Cataract Refract Surg* 1991;17:163–167.

34. Lindquist TD, McGlothan JS, Rotkis WM, et al: Indications for penetrating keratoplasty, 1980–1988. *Cornea* 1991;10:210–216.

35. Haamann P, Jensen OM, Schmidt P: Changing indications for penetrating keratoplasty. *Acta Ophthalmol (Copenh)* 1994;72:443–446.

36. Cursiefen C, Kuchle M, Naumann GO: Changing indications for penetrating keratoplasty: histopathology of 1,250 corneal buttons. *Cornea* 1998;17:468–470.

37. Ramsay AS, Lee WR, Mohammed A: Changing indications for penetrating keratoplasty in the west of Scotland from 1970 to 1995. *Eye* 1997; 11:357–360.

38. Legeais JM, Labetoulle M, Renard G, et al: [Indications for penetrating keratoplasty: a retrospective study of 2,962 cases over 11 years.] *J Fr Ophthalmol* 1993;16:516–522.

39. Price FW Jr, Whitson WE, Marks RG: Graft survival in four common groups of patients undergoing penetrating keratoplasty. *Ophthalmology* 1991;98:322–328.

40. Pineros OE, Cohen EJ, Rapuano CJ, et al: Long-term results after penetrating keratoplasty for Fuchs' endothelial dystrophy. *Arch Ophthalmol* 1996;114:15–18.

41. Olsen T, Ehlers N, Favini E: Long term results of corneal grafting in Fuchs' endothelial dystrophy. *Acta Ophthalmol (Copenh)* 1984;62: 445–452.

42. Stocker FW, Irish A: Fate of successful corneal grafts in Fuchs' endothelial dystrophy. *Am J Ophthalmol* 1969;68:824.

43. Pineros OE, Cohen EJ, Rapuano CJ, et al: Triple vs nonsimultaneous procedures in Fuchs' dystrophy and cataract. *Arch Ophthalmol* 1996; 114:525–528.

44. Payant JA, Gordon LW, VanderZwaag R, et al: Cataract formation following corneal transplantation in eyes with Fuchs' endothelial dystrophy. *Cornea* 1990;9:286–289.

45. al Faran MF, Tabbara KF: Corneal dystrophies among patients undergoing keratoplasty in Saudi Arabia. *Cornea* 1991;10:13–16.

46. Judisch GF, Maumenee IH: Clinical differentiation of recessive congenital hereditary endothelial dystrophy and dominant hereditary endothelial dystrophy. *Am J Ophthalmol* 1978;85: 606–612.

47. Hand CK, Harmon DL, Kennedy SM, et al: Localization of the gene for autosomal recessive congenital hereditary endothelial dystrophy (CHED2) to chromosome 20 by homozygosity mapping. *Genomics* 1999;61:1–4.

48. Callaghan M, Hand CK, Kennedy SM, et al: Homozygosity mapping and linkage analysis demonstrate that autosomal recessive congenital hereditary endothelial dystrophy (CHED) and autosomal dominant CHED are genetically distinct. *Br J Ophthalmol* 1999;83:115–119.

49. Klintworth GK: Advances in the molecular genetics of corneal dystrophies. *Am J Ophthalmol* 1999;128:747–754.

50. Kanis AB, al-Rajhi AA, Taylor CM, et al: Exclusion of AR-CHED from the chromosome 20 region containing the PPMD and AD-CHED loci. *Ophthalmic Genet* 1999;20:243–249.

51. Ehlers N, Modis L, Moller-Pedersen T: A morphological and functional study of congenital hereditary endothelial dystrophy. *Acta Ophthalmol Scand* 1998;76:314–318.

52. Stainer GA, Akers PH, Binder PS, et al: Correlative microscopy and tissue culture of congenital hereditary endothelial dystrophy. *Am J Ophthalmol* 1982;93:456–465.

53. Collum LM, Lavin J, Mullaney J: Congenital hereditary endothelial dystrophy. *Bull Soc Belge Ophtalmol* 1984;211:1–5.

54. McCartney AC, Kirkness CM: Comparison between posterior polymorphous dystrophy and congenital hereditary endothelial dystrophy of the cornea. *Eye* 1988;2:63–70.

55. Daus W, Volcker HE, Homberg A: [Cytology of the corneal endothelium in endothelial dystrophy.] *Fortschr Ophthalmol* 1990;87:364–368.

56. Sekundo W, Marshall GE, Lee WR, et al: Immuno-electron labelling of matrix components in congenital hereditary endothelial dystrophy. *Graefes Arch Clin Exp Ophthalmol* 1994; 232:337–346.

57. Kenyon KR, Antine B: The pathogenesis of congenital hereditary endothelial dystrophy of the cornea. *Am J Ophthalmol* 1971;72:787–795.

58. Kenyon KR, Maumenee AE: Further studies of congenital hereditary endothelial dystrophy of the cornea. *Am J Ophthalmol* 1973;76:419–439.

59. Pedersen OO, Rushood A, Olsen EG: Anterior mesenchymal dysgenesis of the eye: congenital hereditary endothelial dystrophy and congenital glaucoma. *Acta Ophthalmol (Copenh)* 1989;67:470–476.

60. Mullaney PB, Risco JM, Teichmann K, et al: Congenital hereditary endothelial dystrophy associated with glaucoma. *Ophthalmology* 1995;102: 186–192.

61. Pearce WG, Tripathi RC, Morgan G: Congenital endothelial corneal dystrophy: clinical, pathological, and genetic study. *Br J Ophthalmol* 1969;53:577–591.

62. Levenson JE, Chandler JW, Kaufman HE: Affected asymptomatic relatives in congenital hereditary endothelial dystrophy. *Am J Ophthalmol* 1973;76:967–971.

63. Maumenee AE: Congenital hereditary corneal dystrophy. *Am J Ophthalmol* 1960;50: 1114–1124.

64. Sajjadi H, Javadi MA, Hemmati R, et al: Results of penetrating keratoplasty in CHED: congenital hereditary endothelial dystrophy. *Cornea* 1995;14:18–25.

65. al-Rajhi AA, Wagoner MD: Penetrating keratoplasty in congenital hereditary endothelial dystrophy. *Ophthalmology* 1997;104:956–961.

66. Schaumberg DA, Moyes AL, Gomes JA, et al: Corneal transplantation in young children with congenital hereditary endothelial dystrophy. Multicenter Pediatric Keratoplasty Study. *Am J Ophthalmol* 1999;127:373–378.

67. Groh MJ, Gusek-Schneider GC, Seitz B, et al: [Outcomes after penetrating keratoplasty in congenital hereditary corneal endothelial dystrophy (CHED): report on 13 eyes.] *Klin Monatsbl Augenheilkd* 1998;213:201–206.

68. Krachmer JH: Posterior polymorphous corneal dystrophy: a disease characterized by epithelial-like endothelial cells which influence management and prognosis. *Trans Am Ophthalmol Soc* 1985;83:413–475.

69. Koeppe L: [Clinical observations with the slit lamp and the corneal microscope.] *Albrecht von Graefes Arch Klin Exp Ophthalmol* 1916;91: 363–379.

70. Héon E, Mathers WD, Alward WL, et al: Linkage of posterior polymorphous corneal dystrophy to 20q11. *Hum Mol Genet* 1995;4:485–488.

71. Presberg SE, Quigley HA, Forster RK, et al: Posterior polymorphous corneal dystrophy. *Cornea* 1986;4:239–248.

72. Richardson WP, Hettinger ME: Endothelial and epithelial-like cell formations in a case of posterior polymorphous dystrophy. *Arch Ophthalmol* 1985;103:1520–1524.

73. Polack FM, Bourne WM, Forstot SL, et al: Scanning electron microscopy of posterior polymorphous corneal dystrophy. *Am J Ophthalmol* 1980;89:575–584.

74. Rodrigues MM, Sun TT, Krachmer J, et al: Epithelialization of the corneal endothelium in posterior polymorphous dystrophy. *Invest Ophthalmol Vis Sci* 1980;19:832–835.

75. Boruchoff SA, Kuwabara T: Electron microscopy of posterior polymorphous degeneration. *Am J Ophthalmol* 1971;72:879–887.

76. Henriquez AS, Kenyon KR, Dohlman CH, et al: Morphologic characteristics of posterior polymorphous dystrophy: a study of nine corneas and review of the literature. *Surv Ophthalmol* 1984;29:139–147.

77. Rodrigues MM, Waring GO, Laibson PR, et al: Endothelial alterations in congenital corneal dystrophies. *Am J Ophthalmol* 1975;80:678–689.

78. Cibis GW, Tripathi RC: The differential diagnosis of Descemet's tears (Haab's striae) and posterior polymorphous dystrophy bands: a clinicopathologic study. *Ophthalmology* 1982;89: 614–620.

79. Waring GO III, Rodrigues MM, Laibson PR: Corneal dystrophies, II: endothelial dystrophies. *Surv Ophthalmol* 1978;23:147–168.

80. Murphy C, Alvarado J, Juster R: Prenatal and postnatal growth of the human Descemet's membrane. *Invest Ophthalmol Vis Sci* 1984;25: 1402–1415.

81. Cibis GW, Krachmer JA, Phelps CD, et al: The clinical spectrum of posterior polymorphous dystrophy. *Arch Ophthalmol* 1977;95:1529–1537.

82. Laganowski HC, Sherrard ES, Muir MG, et al: Distinguishing features of the iridocorneal endothelial syndrome and posterior polymorphous dystrophy: value of endothelial specular microscopy. *Br J Ophthalmol* 1991;75:212–216.

83. Pratt AW, Saheb NE, Leblanc R: Posterior polymorphous corneal dystrophy and juvenile glaucoma: a case report and brief review of the literature. *Can J Ophthalmol* 1976;11:180–185.

84. Rubenstein RA, Silverman JJ: Hereditary deep dystrophy of the cornea associated with glaucoma and ruptures in Descemet's membrane. *Arch Ophthalmol* 1968;79:123–126.

85. Rodrigues MM, Phelps CD, Krachmer JH, et al: Glaucoma due to endothelialization of the anterior chamber angle: a comparison of posterior polymorphous dystrophy of the cornea and Chandler's syndrome. *Arch Ophthalmol* 1980;98: 688–696.

86. Cibis GW, Krachmer JH, Phelps CD, et al: Iridocorneal adhesions in posterior polymorphous dystrophy. *Trans Am Acad Ophthalmol Otolaryngol* 1976;81:770–777.

87. Bourgeois J, Shields MB, Thresher R: Open angle glaucoma associated with posterior polymorphous dystrophy: a clincopathologic study. *Ophthalmology* 1984;91:420–423.

88. Hirst LW: Congenital anterior segment epithelialisation (case). *Aust J Ophthalmol* 1983;11: 209–213.

89. Grayson M: The nature of hereditary deep polymorphous dystrophy of the cornea: its association with iris and anterior chamber dysgenesis. *Trans Am Ophthalmol Soc* 1974;72:516–559.

90. Hogan MJ, Bietti G: Hereditary deep dystrophy of the cornea (polymorphous). *Am J Ophthalmol* 1968;65:777–788.

91. Driver PJ, Reed JW, Davis RM: Familial cases of keratoconus associated with posterior polymorphous dystrophy. *Am J Ophthalmol* 1994; 118:256–257.

92. Weissman BA, Ehrlich M, Levenson JE, et al: Four cases of keratoconus and posterior polymorphous corneal dystrophy. *Optom Vis Sci* 1989; 66:243–246.

93. Gasset AR, Zimmerman TJ: Posterior polymorphous dystrophy associated with keratoconus. *Am J Ophthalmol* 1974;78:535–537.

94. Molia LM, Lanier JD, Font RL: Posterior polymorphous dystrophy associated with posterior amyloid degeneration of the cornea. *Am J Ophthalmol* 1999;127:86–88.

95. Wagoner MD, Teichmann KD: Terrien's marginal degeneration associated with posterior polymorphous dystrophy. *Cornea* 1999;18: 612–615.

96. Teekhasaenee C, Nimmanit S, Wutthiphan S, et al: Posterior polymorphous dystrophy and Alport syndrome. *Ophthalmology* 1991; 98:1207–1215.

97. Kaiser-Kupfer M, Kuwabara T, Kupfer C: Progressive bilateral essential iris atrophy. *Am J Ophthalmol* 1977;83:340–346.

98. Kupfer C, Kaiser-Kupfer MI, Datiles M, et al: The contralateral eye in the iridocorneal endothelial (ICE) syndrome. *Ophthalmology* 1983; 90:1343–1350.

99. Hemady RK, Patel A, Blum S, et al: Bilateral iridocorneal endothelial syndrome: case report and review of the literature. *Cornea* 1994;13: 368–372.

100. Huna R, Barak A, Melamed S: Bilateral iridocorneal endothelial syndrome presented as Cogan-Reese and Chandler's syndrome. *J Glaucoma* 1996;5:60–62.

101. Teekhasaenee C, Ritch R: Iridocorneal endothelial syndrome in Thai patients: clinical variations. *Arch Ophthalmol* 2000;118:187–192.

102. Sherrard ES, Frangoulis MA, Muir MG: On the morphology of cells of posterior cornea in the iridocorneal endothelial syndrome. *Cornea* 1991;10:233–243.

103. Sekundo W, Lee WR, Kirkness CM, et al: An ultrastructural investigation of an early manifestation of the posterior polymorphous dystrophy of the cornea. *Ophthalmology* 1994;101: 1422–1431.

104. Yanoff M: Iridocorneal endothelial syndrome: unification of a disease spectrum. *Surv Ophthalmol* 1979;24:1–2.

105. Eagle RC Jr, Font RL, Yanoff M, et al: Proliferative endotheliopathy with iris abnormalities: the iridocorneal endothelial syndrome. *Arch Ophthalmol* 1979;97:2104–2111.

106. Shields MB: Progressive essential iris atrophy, Chandler's syndrome, and the iris nevus (Cogan-Reese) syndrome: a spectrum of disease. *Surv Ophthalmol* 1979;24:3–20.

107. Langova A, Praznovska Z, Farkasova B: [Progressive essential atrophy of the iris as a form of the iridocorneal endothelial (ICE) syndrome.] *Cesk Slov Oftalmol* 1997;53:371–380.

108. Harms C: [Unilateral spontaneous rupture formation of the iris during atrophy without mechanical stress.] *Klin Monatsbl Augenheilkd* 1903;41:522.

109. Chandler PA: Atrophy of the stroma of the iris: endothelial dystrophy, corneal edema, and glaucoma. *Am J Ophthalmol* 1956;41:607.

110. Cogan DG, Reese AB: A syndrome of iris nodules, ectopic Descemet's membrane, and unilateral glaucoma. *Arch Ophthalmol* 1975;93: 963.

111. Alvarado JA, Underwood JL, Green WR, et al: Detection of herpes simplex viral DNA in the iridocorneal endothelial syndrome. *Arch Ophthalmol* 1994;112:1601–1609.

112. Groh MJ, Seitz B, Schumacher S, et al: Detection of herpes simplex virus in aqueous humor in iridocorneal endothelial (ICE) syndrome. *Cornea* 1999;18:359–360.

113. Howell DN, Damms T, Burchette JL Jr, et al: Endothelial metaplasia in the iridocorneal endothelial syndrome. *Invest Ophthalmol Vis Sci* 1997;38:1896–1901.

114. Hirst LW, Bancroft J, Yamauchi K, et al: Immunohistochemical pathology of the corneal endothelium in iridocorneal endothelial syndrome. *Invest Ophthalmol Vis Sci* 1995;36:820–827.

115. Bahn CF, Falls HF, Varley GA, et al: Classification of corneal endothelial disorders based on neural crest origin. *Ophthalmology* 1984;91: 558–563.

116. Crawford GJ, Stulting RD, Cavanagh HD, et al: Penetrating keratoplasty in the management of iridocorneal endothelial syndrome. *Cornea* 1989;8:34–40.

117. Bourne WM: Partial corneal involvement in the iridocorneal endothelial syndrome. *Am J Ophthalmol* 1982;94:774–781.

118. Blum JV, Allen JH, Holland MG: Familial bilateral essential iris atrophy (group 2). *Trans Am Acad Ophthalmol Otolaryngol* 1962;66: 493–500.

119. Jampol LM, Rosser MJ, Sears ML: Unusual aspects of progressive essential iris atrophy. *Am J Ophthalmol* 1974;77:353–357.

120. Hirst LW: Bilateral iridocorneal endothelial syndrome. *Cornea* 1995;14:331.

121. Quigley HA, Forster RF: Histopathology of cornea and iris in Chandler's syndrome. *Arch Ophthalmol* 1978;96:1878–1882.

122. Bourne WM, Brubaker RF: Decreased endothelial permeability in the iridocorneal endothelial syndrome. *Ophthalmology* 1982;89: 591–595.

123. Hirst LW, Green WR, Luckenbach M, et al: Epithelial characteristics of the endothelium in Chandler's syndrome. *Invest Ophthalmol Vis Sci* 1983;24:603–611.

124. Portis JM, Stamper RL, Spencer WH, et al: The corneal endothelium and Descemet's membrane in the iridocorneal endothelial syndrome. *Trans Am Ophthalmol Soc* 1985;83:316–331.

125. Chiou AG, Kaufman SC, Beuerman RW, et al: Confocal microscopy in the iridocorneal endothelial syndrome. *Br J Ophthalmol* 1999;83: 697–702.

126. Levy SG, Moss J, Sawada H, et al: The composition of wide-spaced collagen in normal and diseased Descemet's membrane. *Curr Eye Res* 1996;15:45–52.

127. Levy SG, McCartney AC, Sawada H, et al: Descemet's membrane in the iridocorneal-endothelial syndrome: morphology and composition. *Exp Eye Res* 1995;61:323–333.

128. Levy SG, McCartney AC, Bagli MH, et al: Pathology of the iridocorneal-endothelial syndrome: the ICE-cell. *Invest Ophthalmol Vis Sci* 1995;36:2592–2601.

129. Levy SG, Kirkness CM, Moss J, et al: The histopathology of the iridocorneal-endothelial syndrome. *Cornea* 1996;15:46–54.

130. Shields MB, Campbell DG, Simmons RJ: The essential iris atrophies. *Am J Ophthalmol* 1978;85:749–759.

131. Chang PC, Soong HK, Couto MF, et al: Prognosis for penetrating keratoplasty in iridocorneal endothelial syndrome. *Refract Corneal Surg* 1993;9:129–132.

132. Fulcher S, Lui GM, Houston LL, et al: Use of immunotoxin to inhibit proliferating human corneal endothelium. *Invest Ophthalmol Vis Sci* 1988;29:755–759.

133. Shields MB: *Textbook of Glaucoma.* 2nd ed. Baltimore, MD: Williams & Wilkins; 1987.

134. Assaad MH, Baerveldt G, Rockwood EJ: Glaucoma drainage devices: pros and cons. *Curr Opin Ophthalmol* 1999;10:147–153.

135. Eagle RC Jr, Font RL, Yanoff M, et al: The iris naevus (Cogan-Reese) syndrome: light and electron microscopic observations. *Br J Ophthalmol* 1980;64:446–452.

136. Ye T, Pang Y, Liu Y: Iris nevus syndrome (report of 9 cases). *Eye Sci* 1991;7:34–39.

137. Kidd M, Hetherington J, Magee S: Surgical results in iridocorneal endothelial syndrome. *Arch Ophthalmol* 1988;106:199–201.

138. Lanzl IM, Wilson RP, Dudley D, et al: Outcome of trabeculectomy with mitomycin-C in the iridocorneal endothelial syndrome. *Ophthalmology* 2000;107:295–297.

139. Kim DK, Aslanides IM, Schmidt CM Jr, et al: Long-term outcome of aqueous shunt surgery in ten patients with iridocorneal endothelial syndrome. *Ophthalmology* 1999;106:1030–1034.

140. Chen J, Liu Z, Yu L: [Corneal endothelial decompensation of iridocorneal endothelial syndrome treated by penetrating keratoplasty.] *Chung Hua Yen Ko Tsa Chih* 1996;32:264–266.

141. Buxton JN, Lash RS: Results of penetrating keratoplasty in the iridocorneal endothelial syndrome. *Am J Ophthalmol* 1984;98:297–301.

142. DeBroff BM, Thoft RA: Surgical results of penetrating keratoplasty in essential iris atrophy. *J Refract Corneal Surg* 1994;10:428–432.

CHAPTER 5

Corneal and Conjunctival Degenerations

Beth A. Handwerger, MD
Christopher J. Rapuano, MD
Ming X. Wang, MD, PhD
Peter R. Laibson, MD

Corneal degenerations consist of abnormal deposits or structural changes in the cornea that have been distinguished from corneal dystrophies. Corneal degenerations tend to be unilateral, but are often bilateral and occur sporadically. Many degenerations are considered changes associated with aging, because they appear later in life. Progression varies, but can be rapid. The peripheral cornea is affected more often than the central cornea; thus, vision is less likely to be impaired than with the dystrophies. Local and systemic diseases are commonly associated with corneal degenerations. These degenerations can occur in the presence of other eye abnormalities, such as inflammation and neovascularization.[1,2]

In contrast, corneal dystrophies are typically bilateral, symmetric, noninflammatory, and hereditary. They appear earlier in life and progress slowly. The central cornea is usually involved, resulting in visual symptoms. Systemic diseases are not generally associated with corneal dystrophies.

5-1

AGE-RELATED CORNEAL DEGENERATIONS

5-1-1 Arcus Senilis

Arcus senilis, also known as *circulus senilis* or *corneal arcus*, is the deposition of lipid in the peripheral corneal stroma (Figure 5-1). It is a bilateral degenerative process. Lipid deposits are first seen near Descemet's membrane and later near Bowman's layer. The opacity extends through the stroma in an hourglass fashion, as demonstrated on histopathology. Arcus forms in the inferior cornea first, then in the superior cornea, and later nasally and temporally to form a complete ring or circle. The borders of arcus are sharper peripherally than centrally.[1,2]

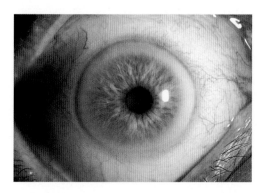

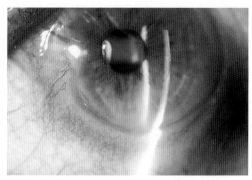

Figure 5-1 *Arcus senilis. Deposition of lipid, sparing rim of peripheral cornea. First started as arc above and below and later extended to 360°.*

Figure 5-2 *Furrow degeneration in arcus senilis. Peripheral thinning as seen in slit-lamp view. This patient had one third thinning of peripheral cornea in quiet eye, which remained stable for years.*

A clear zone exists between the limbus and the lipid deposition in the cornea. Thinning that occurs in this clear zone is called *furrow degeneration* (Figure 5-2). This thinning is not a risk for visual loss, inflammation, vascularization, or perforation. Patients with arcus senilis and furrow degeneration are asymptomatic.

Arcus senilis is common: 60% of men between the ages of 40 and 60 have it, and almost 100% of men over 80 years old have it. In women, arcus occurs later, and in African Americans, it occurs earlier.

In patients less than 40 years old, arcus is an indication for laboratory testing because it may occur with lipid abnormalities, such as hyperlipoproteinemia and hypercholesterolemia. Nephrotic syndrome, hypothyroidism, high cholesterol intake, obstructive jaundice, and diabetic ketoacidosis may increase the level of lipoproteins and cause corneal arcus. Unilateral arcus may be an indication of carotid artery disease. The eye without arcus is the side where the carotid disease may be more severe.

5-1-2 Hassall-Henle Bodies

Hassall-Henle bodies, or Descemet's warts, are small localized excrescences of Descemet's membrane in the peripheral cornea.[1,2] These bodies represent a normal aging change resulting from an overproduction of basement membrane by peripheral endothelial cells. The collagenous structure is the same as normal Descemet's membrane. Specular reflection is the best method to identify these dark round holes, which are analogous to the cornea guttata that occurs centrally. On histopathology, Hassall-Henle bodies are identical to the central cornea guttata of endothelial dystrophy, except that progressive endothelial damage does not occur. Hassall-Henle bodies are rarely found in patients younger than 25 years old. They increase in number as a person ages. Patients with Hassall-Henle bodies are asymptomatic.

5-1-3 Limbal Girdle of Vogt

The limbal girdle of Vogt is a bilateral yellow-white band at the nasal and temporal limbus of the peripheral cornea.[1,2] When exposure occurs, the inferior limbus may be involved as well. The incidence of the limbal girdle increases with age. It is asymptomatic and requires no treatment. Traditionally, there are two types:

1. Type 1 is characterized by a well-demarcated white band that may have holes. A clear area is adjacent to the limbus, and there is a sharp border centrally (Figure 5-3). This opacity is thought to represent early calcific band keratopathy.

2. Type 2 is a solid chalky band, without either holes or a clear zone near the limbus, that may extend centrally in an irregular linear fashion.

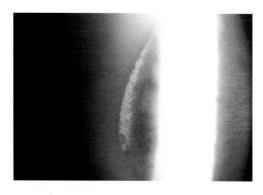

Figure 5-3 *Limbal girdle of Vogt. Note thin whitish yellow band at temporal limbus, with clear rim of cornea between band and limbus. This band did not extend superiorly and inferiorly. It represents elastotic degeneration similar to that seen in pterygium and pinguecula.*

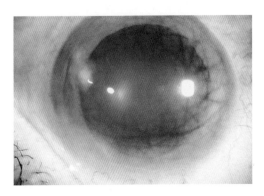

Figure 5-4 *Crocodile shagreen. Appearance of "crocodile leather," with patchy areas of stromal opacity separated by lucent lines. This posterior crocodile shagreen is solely an age-related change.*

The limbal girdle of Vogt can be visualized using direct illumination, although the best method combines retroillumination and sclerotic scatter. On histopathology, the lesion is subepithelial and may have overlying epithelial atrophy. Calcification at the level of Bowman's layer and elastotic changes, as seen in pterygium and pinguecula, have been identified.

5-1-4 Crocodile Shagreen

Crocodile shagreen is an area of cobblestone or crocodile-skin appearance in the anterior or posterior cornea.[3] Polygonal gray-to-white opacities form and are separated by lucent lines (Figure 5-4). This degeneration is usually bilateral and is not visually significant. No treatment is indicated. On histopathology, stromal folds are seen near Bowman's layer in the anterior form and near Descemet's membrane in the posterior form. Irregularly arranged collagen in a sawtooth pattern is found in the grayish opacity, with calcium deposits at some of the peaks.

Anterior crocodile shagreen may be an aging change, although similar changes can be seen in trauma, band keratopathy, hypotony, juvenile X-linked megalocornea, and keratoconus patients wearing hard contact lenses. Posterior crocodile shagreen is solely an age-related change.

5-1-5 Cornea Farinata

Cornea farinata is an asymptomatic corneal degeneration characterized by very fine opacities in the posterior stroma, best seen by retroillumination off the iris. *Farinata*, from the Latin *farina*, meaning "flour," is an apt name for these opacities, which resemble flour in size and color. They do not affect vision. On histopathology, a lipofuscin-like material is found in the vacuoles of posterior stromal keratocytes.

5-1-6 Polymorphic Amyloid Degeneration

Polymorphic amyloid degeneration is a bilateral and localized degenerative form of amyloid deposition in the cornea that is not heritable or associated with any other disease.[3] Patients are usually at least 50 years old. Polymorphic punctate or filamentous opacities are found throughout the stroma, usually in the central cornea. These deposits can occur as dots, commas, single lines, or branching lines similar to lattice dystrophy (Figure 5-5). On direct illumination, the lesions appear gray, whereas on retroillumination, they appear refractile and clear. No treatment is necessary, as the deposits do not cause visual symptoms. Histopathologically, the deposits are consistent with amyloid.

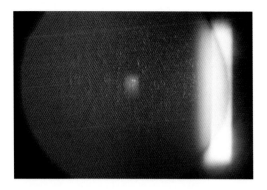

Figure 5-5 *Polymorphic amyloid degeneration. These lesions are very hard to see, as they are fine and usually in mid-to-deep stroma. They are seen best on retroillumination, as pictured here.*

5-2

NON–AGE-RELATED CORNEAL DEGENERATIONS

5-2-1 Band Keratopathy

Subepithelial calcium deposits in Bowman's layer are called *band keratopathy* or *calcific degeneration*. Commonly, this keratopathy is associated with chronic ocular inflammatory disease, such as uveitis, interstitial keratitis, or hypercalcemic states, such as renal failure and hyperphosphatemia (Figure 5-6 and Table 5-1). It can occur secondary to topical medication use. Band keratopathy

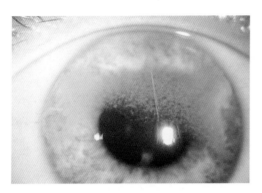

Figure 5-6 *Band keratopathy. This patient had chronic uveitis in childhood and continues to have 3+ flare and occasional cells. Patient developed calcium in periphery, which then crossed central cornea in band shape. Condition responded to medical removal with disodium EDTA, leaving patient with clear central cornea and only peripheral calcium deposits.*

TABLE 5-1

Common Causes of Band Keratopathy

Chronic ocular disease
    Interstitial keratitis
    Prolonged keratitis or corneal edema
    Phthisis
    Chronic uveitis

Hypercalcemia caused by
    Hyperparathyroidism
    Sarcoidosis
    Vitamin D toxicity
    Milk–alkali syndrome

Hyperphosphatemia with normal calcium
(in some patients with renal failure)

Intraocular silicone oil (aphakic eye)

Chemical exposure in ophthalmic medications
(mercury)

Keratoconjunctivitis sicca

Systemic disease

Primary hereditary band keratopathy

Idiopathic

usually starts as a gray-white opacity in the nasal and temporal interpalpebral zone and advances centrally, with continued chronic ocular inflammation (Figure 5-7). The band is well demarcated at the peripheral edge by a lucent zone, whereas the central edge fades into normal cornea. Often, there are Swiss cheese–like holes in the band.

Band keratopathy progresses slowly over months to years. However, in severe keratoconjunctivitis sicca, significant calcium deposition can occur over weeks. With most patients, the cause of the condition is known. If the cause is not known by history or ocular examination, a medical evaluation, including serum calcium, phosphorus, uric acid, and renal function measurements, is indicated. If hyperparathyroidism or sarcoidosis is suspected, parathyroid hormone (PTH) and angiotensin-converting enzyme (ACE) testing should be performed.

Generally, patients with band keratopathy are asymptomatic, unless the band extends into the visual axis, causing decreased vision, or the band involves the corneal epithelium or flakes off, causing irritation and foreign body sensation (Figure 5-8). Some patients complain of painful recurrent erosions and a poor cosmetic appearance.

If symptoms become severe, treatment for band keratopathy is indicated to remove or reduce the calcification. After any possible systemic or ocular causes are treated, the first line of therapy is lubrication to decrease discomfort. Occasionally, thick flaking calcium can be scraped or removed with a blade and forceps under topical anesthesia. The mainstay of treatment consists of removal of overlying epithelium under topical anesthesia, followed by calcium chelation with disodium ethylenediaminetetraacetic acid (Na-EDTA). Na-EDTA of 0.05 molar concentration is diluted 1:3 with sterile saline and applied directly to the calcium on saturated cellulose sponges or cotton-tipped applicators. This procedure may take 10 to 45 minutes, depending on the severity of the calcium deposition. Excimer laser phototherapeutic keratectomy can be used to treat residual anterior corneal haze after Na-EDTA chelation.[4]

Band keratopathy may recur, especially if the underlying causative condition persists. Phototherapeutic keratectomy is usually not employed as primary treatment for calcific degeneration, because it is expensive and may not be as effective as chelation for central superficial band keratopathy.

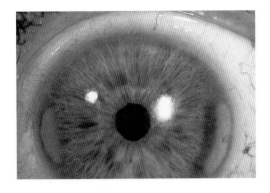

Figure 5-7 *Band keratopathy. In this patient, band keratopathy started in periphery nasally and temporally and remained in this area for many years.*

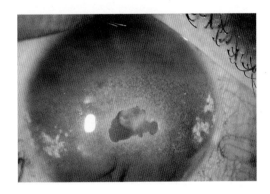

Figure 5-8 *Band keratopathy. In this patient, band keratopathy extends across central cornea, with area of clearing. Note very sharp light reflex, indicating smooth anterior corneal surface. Band keratopathy is in region of Bowman's layer.*

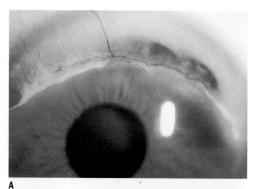

A

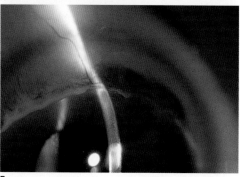

B

Figure 5-9 *Terrien marginal degeneration. (A) Thinning in superior cornea at periphery, with lipid deposits in bed of lesion and at central corneal edge. In most cases, thinning does not progress to perforation. Lesions may progress circumferentially or they may remain stationary. (B) Peripheral thinning as seen with slit lamp in same patient.*

5-2-2 Terrien Marginal Degeneration

Terrien marginal degeneration is a slowly progressive peripheral corneal inflammatory and degenerative disorder.[1,2] This degeneration is rare and the cause is not known. Men are affected more than women by a 3:1 ratio. It can occur at any age, but rarely in the first decade and most commonly between 20 and 40 years of age. The condition is bilateral, although the second eye may be affected decades later.

The degenerative process generally starts in the supranasal peripheral cornea, with small white opacities in the anterior stroma. Overlying superficial vascularization occurs, and later the peripheral cornea thins under an intact epithelium. The thinned corneal arc becomes more vascularized and wider over time. The thinning may extend centrally or circumferentially. Lipid deposits are seen in the advancing edge of the gutter (Figures 5-9 and 5-10).

The condition presents in two different forms:

1. Younger patients tend to have more of an inflammatory Terrien degeneration, with recurrent inflammatory episodes of episcleritis and scleritis. Topical corticosteroids may be used as treatment.

2. In older patients, the degenerative form is more common. It progresses more slowly and patients remain asymptomatic for many years.

Patients become symptomatic when their vision suffers from increased astigmatism. Terrien marginal degeneration is characterized by against-the-rule astigmatism, resulting from the superior or inferior marginal thinning.

The histopathology is variable, with a normal, thin, or thick epithelium. Bowman's layer may be fragmented or absent, and Descemet's membrane may have breaks in the thinned areas. With severe thinning, aqueous can connect to the subepithelial space, resulting in a filtering bleb and hypotony. Histiocytes found in the pathologic specimen are filled with collagen breakdown products. Inflammatory cells may be present.

There is no known method to prevent Terrien marginal degeneration. Patients' symptoms can often be alleviated with astigmatism correction in spectacles or contact lenses. If the cornea thins severely to the point at which perforation is at risk or in cases of very high astigmatism, a lamellar or eccentric lamellar penetrating keratoplasty may be performed. Perforation may occur spontaneously or as the result of minor trauma in 15% of patients.

5-2-3 Spheroidal Degeneration

Spheroidal degeneration refers to a degenerative condition that can occur in the cornea and conjunctiva.[1,2] Other names for this entity include *climatic droplet keratopathy, Labrador keratopathy, corneal elastosis, fisherman's keratitis, keratinoid corneal degeneration,* and *chronic actinic keratopathy.*

Spheroidal degeneration may occur as a primary condition in the cornea, without any other ocular disease, or as a secondary manifestation from ocular inflammation or injury. This degenerative process can occur in the conjunctiva alone or in association with the corneal condition. Ultraviolet exposure, aging, and environmental trauma are major factors contributing to the devel-

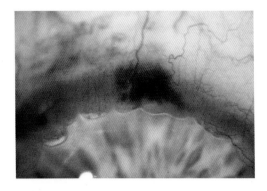

Figure 5-10 *Terrien marginal degeneration. Hemorrhage in bed gradually healed without further thinning. In this patient, lipid deposit is at central corneal edge, indicating slow progression. Lipid is deposited from leading edge of capillaries in thinned bed. Patient was comfortable and central vision was good, as peripheral thinning did not cause significant astigmatism.*

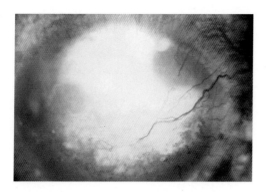

Figure 5-11 *Spheroidal degeneration. Large golden-brown elevated spherules with vascularization can be seen in inferior part of cornea.*
Courtesy Resident Slide Collection, Wills Eye Hospital, 1996.

opment of this condition. Men are affected more than women, possibly because of occupation-related exposure. Corneal neo-vascularization, herpetic infection, glaucoma, and lattice corneal dystrophy have been associated with secondary spheroidal degeneration.

Spheroidal degeneration begins typically with clumps of small clear droplets under the epithelium of the cornea, conjunctiva, or both in the interpalpebral zone at the 3- and 9-o'clock positions. As the degeneration progresses, the spherules enlarge, become gold or brown, and progress centrally. They can coalesce into larger droplets and become elevated (Figure 5-11).

Histopathology reveals protein deposits in the extracellular space. Abnormal collagen fibers adjacent to spherules are seen on electron microscopy. Both of these changes are also characteristics of the elastotic degeneration seen in pterygium and pinguecula.

Usually, patients are asymptomatic, unless the visual axis contains spherules, resulting in decreased vision. Advanced lesions may become nodular and break through the epithelium, causing irritation. Conjunctival lesions can be excised directly. Excimer laser phototherapeutic, lamellar, or penetrating keratoplasty may be indicated when vision is affected.

5-2-4 Salzmann Nodular Degeneration

Salzmann nodular degeneration typically occurs in eyes that have, or have had, chronic inflammation.[5] The process occurs in association with many diseases, including interstitial keratitis, herpetic keratitis, vernal keratoconjunctivitis, trachoma, phlyctenular disease, and keratoconjunctivitis sicca. It

TABLE 5-2

Conditions Associated With
Salzmann Nodular Degeneration

Inflammatory

Interstitial keratitis

Chalazion

Vernal keratoconjunctivitis

Trachoma

Phlyctenular keratitis

Noninflammatory

Postoperative corneal surgery

Filamentary keratitis

Basement membrane dystrophy

Hard contact lenses

Keratoconus

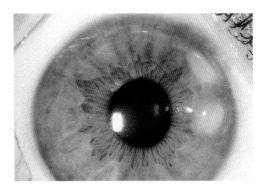

Figure 5-12 *Salzmann nodular degeneration. Two elevated gray-white lesions contain collagen plaques with hyalinization. As these lesions are in periphery, they do not affect central vision. They may remain unchanged for many years or progress very slowly.*

also occurs in noninflammatory conditions, such as epithelial basement membrane dystrophy, following corneal surgery, and occasionally in the absence of corneal disease (Table 5-2).

Salzmann nodular degeneration is characterized by single or multiple white, gray-white, or bluish elevated lesions in the central or peripheral cornea adjacent to an area of corneal scarring, vascularization, edema, or even normal cornea (Figures 5-12 and 5-13). The prevalence increases with aging and is higher in women. Often, the degeneration presents bilaterally. The nodules contain collagen plaques with hyalinization stained with Masson trichrome between the corneal epithelium and stroma. The presence or absence of Bowman's layer under the nodule is variable. Patients are generally asymptomatic, unless the visual axis is

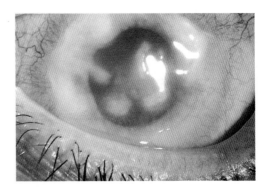

Figure 5-13 *Salzmann nodular degeneration. Progressive changes in central cornea, causing opacification and irregular astigmatism. Note irregular light reflex compared to regular light reflex in Figure 5-8. In this case, superficial keratectomy was able to restore significant vision, as these lesions are usually at or above Bowman's layer.*

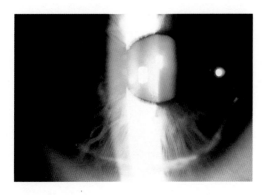

Figure 5-14 *Pellucid marginal degeneration. Crescent-shaped band of thinned cornea can be seen inferiorly, spanning from 4- to 8-o'clock position near limbus. Thinned area is clear and epithelial defect or vascularization is absent.*
Courtesy Resident Slide Collection, Wills Eye Hospital, 1996.

involved or the lesions are considerably elevated. Foreign body sensation and erosions of the epithelium can occur with notably elevated nodules.

Treatment depends on symptoms. For mild irritation, lubrication is the mainstay of therapy. For erosions and visual axis involvement, a superficial keratectomy can be performed. As the lesions are often above Bowman's layer, this layer can be maintained generally. If the lesions extend into the visual axis, a lamellar keratectomy with a blade is frequently beneficial. Less commonly, the excimer laser can also be used to treat lesions that extend into the anterior stroma. For deep stromal disease impairing vision, a lamellar keratoplasty may be indicated. Salzmann nodular degeneration can recur in grafts or after keratectomy.

5-2-5 Pellucid Marginal Degeneration

Pellucid marginal degeneration is a corneal thinning and ectatic condition in which a crescent-shaped band of thinning forms in the inferior portion of the cornea near the limbus, typically spanning from the 4- to the 8-o'clock position. The thinned area is about 1 to 2 mm wide and typically is clear, with no epithelial defect or vascularization (Figure 5-14). In contrast to keratoconus, in which an anteriorly protruded area is below the area of thinning, the protruded area in pellucid marginal degeneration is typically located superior to the thinned band.

Patients with pellucid marginal degeneration typically present at middle age with the complaint of blurred vision uncorrectable with spectacles or contact lenses because of the high against-the-rule astigmatism. There is generally no family history. As with keratoconus, pellucid marginal degeneration can progress over time, with an increased amount of thinning and ectasia; hydrops and corneal scarring can occur. Several common diagnostic signs of keratoconus are typically absent in pellucid marginal degeneration, such as iron line (Fleischer ring) and Vogt's striae.

Histopathologically, pellucid marginal degeneration is characterized by corneal stromal thinning and absence of Bowman's layer in the affected area.[6,7] The treatment of pellucid marginal degeneration is mainly aimed at reducing the large amount of against-the-rule astigmatism caused by the inferior thinning and area of anterior protrusion superior to it. With disease progression, spectacles or contact lenses are often not effective. Surgical treatment for pellucid marginal degeneration includes eccentric lamellar or penetrating graft or resection of the thinned area. These treatments appear to offer both correction of astigmatism and removal of the thinned area.[8] Surgery for pellucid marginal degeneration is, in general, not satisfactory because of the close proximity of the diseased area to the corneal limbus, giving rise to high postoperative complications, such as graft rejection, neovascularization, and astigmatism.

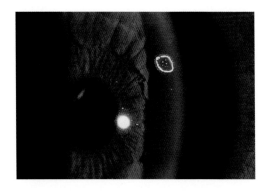

Figure 5-15 *Coats white ring. Coats ring does not distort images, even when over visual axis. This ring, seen at high magnification, is not over visual axis. Lesions are usually quite small; this was one of the larger ones these authors have seen.*

5-2-6 Coats White Ring

Coats white ring is presumably caused by a traumatic injury, usually from a metallic foreign body. A partial or complete white ring 1 mm or less in diameter is formed in the cornea (Figure 5-15). This degeneration is composed of discrete white dots, which may coalesce in Bowman's layer or the anterior stroma. The lesion is asymptomatic and requires no treatment. Histopathology has revealed the presence of iron.

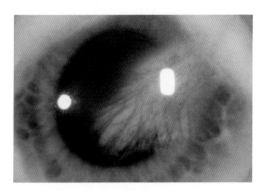

Figure 5-16 *Lipid keratopathy. Note whitish yellow opacities, with lines of clearing where vessels are present. Vessels in this case are quiescent, but can open and have significant blood flow with any recurrent inflammation. Lipid is deposited from leading edge of capillaries as they progress into cornea.*

5-2-7 Lipid Keratopathy

Primary lipid keratopathy is rare and is not associated with trauma, corneal vascularization, or hyperlipidemia. Cholesterol, triglycerides, and phospholipids deposit in the posterior stroma and Descemet's membrane in a similar location as arcus senilis.[1,2] This keratopathy may be caused by increased vascular permeability of limbal blood vessels or extrusions of lipid from abnormal keratocytes. Histopathology demonstrates fewer stromal cells when lipid degeneration is present.

Secondary lipid degeneration is more common and is typically associated with corneal neovascularization occurring with interstitial keratitis, herpetic keratitis (simplex or zoster), trauma, corneal hydrops, corneal ulceration, and hypoxia as a complication of contact lens use. Lipid deposits in the cornea may be caused by increased permeability of the vessels or an inability of the vessels to remove lipid (Figure 5-16). The lipid deposits in the stroma form a gray to yellow-white infiltrate. The characteristic appearance is a sea fan with feathery edges or a dense discoid lesion adjacent to the blood vessels. Active inflammation tends to form a discoid lesion. Inactive neovascularization from old inflammation may deposit lipid in a sea-fan shape. Cholesterol crystals may appear at the edges of the keratopathy.

Lipid keratopathy is difficult to treat successfully. Treating the underlying condition is the most effective method of control. Corneal neovascularization can be managed with topical corticosteroids, which may reduce lipid deposits and prevent progression. Laser therapy to corneal vessels has been performed without consistent long-lasting effect. When vision is compromised from lipid keratopathy, penetrating kerato-plasty may be beneficial; however, the risk of rejection is increased with a vascularized cornea.

5-2-8 Pigmentary Iron Lines

Iron is seen as a yellow to dark-brown dis-coloration in the corneal epithelium in mul-tiple corneal conditions.[9,10] The source and cause of the iron are controversial. Tears may pool on an irregular corneal surface, causing iron to accumulate, or deposits may occur at trauma sites from the change in corneal contour. On histopathology, ferritin is located intracellularly and extracellularly in the basal epithelium of the cornea.

The Hudson-Stähli line, the most com-mon iron line, is found in the normal cornea of individuals of all ages. It is a horizontal line located at the level of the tear menis-cus, in the lower third of the cornea, where the eyelid meets the cornea. Corneal scars and contact lens wear may change the loca-tion or broaden the line. The line becomes more prominent with the passage of time. Typically, it is bilateral and symmetric, al-though it can occur unilaterally or asym-metrically. Individuals are affected from the age of 2, with an increased incidence up to age 70.

Ferry's line is found anterior to a filter-ing bleb following glaucoma surgery. It may be related to the size of the bleb. Stocker's line is located at the advancing edge of a pterygium. Keratoconus patients may have a Fleischer ring at the base of the cone (Table 5-3).

Iron lines have also been seen following traumatic injuries, corneal scars, penetrat-ing keratoplasty,[11] and refractive surgical procedures, including radial keratotomy (Figure 5-17), excimer laser photorefractive

TABLE 5-3

Epithelial Iron Lines

Name	Location
Hudson-Stähli line	Lower one third of cornea above eyelid margin
Fleischer ring	Base of cone in keratoconus
Stocker's line	Head of pterygium
Ferry's line	Anterior to filtering bleb

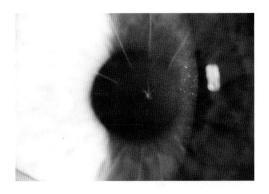

Figure 5-17 *Pigmentary iron line. Deposited between radial keratotomy cuts in central clear cornea, this iron line did not affect central visual acuity. Iron lines at base of cone in keratoconus and at head of pterygium also are quiescent and do not alter vision. They seem to be present where there is some chronic irregularity of corneal surface.*

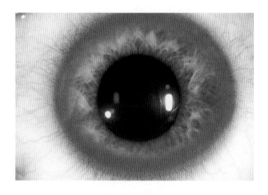

Figure 5-18 *Copper deposit. Kayser-Fleischer ring in patient with abnormal copper metabolism. Ring is usually in peripheral cornea, involving deep stroma and Descemet's membrane.*

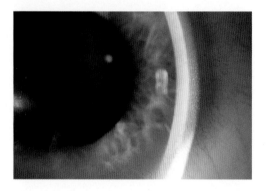

Figure 5-19 *Copper deposit. In this slit-lamp view, note yellowish brown deposits in region of deep stroma and Descemet's membrane, which is typical for Kayser-Fleischer ring.*

keratectomy, and laser-assisted in situ keratomileusis (LASIK). Iron lines can be found adjacent to any corneal irregularity. In radial keratotomy, the iron lines form a stellate pattern in the central cornea.

5-2-9 Corneal Deposits

5-2-9-1 Copper   The accumulation of copper in the eye, called *ocular chalcosis,* or in the body can cause a gray-green or yellow-brown discoloration in Descemet's membrane (Figures 5-18 and 5-19). When associated with systemic copper overload in Wilson disease, the discoloration is called a *Kayser-Fleischer ring.* This ring is found in the peripheral cornea and can be seen by slit lamp when prominent and by gonioscopy when less prominent. Other conditions causing a copper overload, such as chronic active hepatitis, primary biliary cirrhosis, progressive intrahepatic cholestasis, and multiple myeloma, can cause copper deposition in Descemet's membrane. A copper intraocular foreign body can also cause copper deposition in Descemet's membrane. Treatment with penicillamine removes copper from the body and from Descemet's membrane; thus, the success of treatment in Wilson disease can be correlated with a less prominent Kayser-Fleischer ring.

5-2-9-2 Gold   Systemic gold therapy for rheumatoid arthritis can cause gold deposition in the cornea, called *corneal chrysiasis.* Gold deposits in the deep stroma and Descemet's membrane and appears yellow-brown. These deposits are not visually significant and are not an indication to cease treatment. They may be reversible if therapy is discontinued.

5-2-9-3 Silver The deposition of silver in the eye is called *argyrosis*. Argyrol, a topical medication containing silver, was the main cause of this condition in the past. The medication caused a diffuse gray discoloration of the eyelid skin and conjunctiva (Figure 5-20) and a gold-gray discoloration in Descemet's membrane. The deposition did not cause visual symptoms.

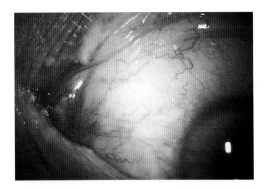

Figure 5-20 *Silver deposit. Argyrosis with grayish pigmentation of conjunctiva, particularly near plica, in patient who used Argyrol for 20 years. Argyrol was commonly used antiseptic before antibiotics became available to treat all kinds of conjunctival inflammations and infections.*

5-3

CONJUNCTIVAL DEGENERATIONS

5-3-1 Pinguecula

A pinguecula (plural: pingueculae) is a gray or white-yellow fleshy-appearing lesion found in the interpalpebral conjunctiva (Figure 5-21). It is typically a bilateral degenerative process found more often in the nasal than temporal conjunctiva, and the incidence increases with age. Actinic exposure, dust, and wind are thought to be predisposing factors for the formation of a pinguecula. In warm climates and in individuals with occupational sun exposure (for example, lifeguards and farmers), the lesion occurs more often. Ultraviolet-protective eyewear may prevent the development of a pinguecula.[1,2]

A pinguecula is typically asymptomatic. Rarely, it may cause a problem with contact lens fitting or cosmesis. Occasionally, inflammation of a pinguecula, called *pingueculitis*, occurs, resulting in redness and irritation or foreign body sensation. The inflammation can be treated topically with lubrication, corticosteroids, or nonsteroidal anti-inflammatory drugs (NSAIDs). Surgical excision is indicated for recurrent or chronic inflammation, contact lens intolerance, or cosmetic

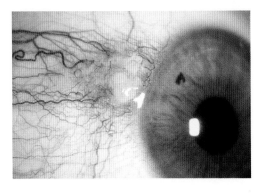

Figure 5-21 *Pinguecula. This pinguecula is fleshy, elevated, and vascularized, but does not invade cornea. Pinguecula may be mild, with few or no vessels, and flat or slightly elevated, as this one is. This inflamed pinguecula caused symptoms of irritation and stained superficially with fluorescein.*

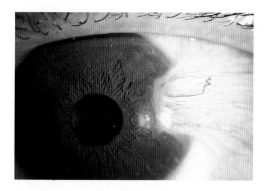

Figure 5-22 *Pterygium. Growing onto cornea from nasal limbus in wing-like configuration, this pterygium caused symptoms of irritation and was cosmetic problem for patient.*

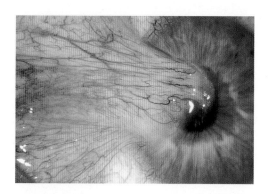

Figure 5-23 *Pterygium. This large recurrent pterygium was accompanied by double vision and discomfort. One problem with pterygium removal is recurrence. Incidence of recurrence is very high, leaving bare sclera, as in this case. Pterygium removal was done again, but this time successfully, with conjunctival transplant.*

concerns. On histopathology, elastotic degeneration of the substantia propria is present, but there is no elastic tissue.

5-3-2 Pterygium

A pterygium (plural: pterygia) is a wing-shaped fibrovascular tissue growth extending from the bulbar conjunctiva onto the cornea (Figures 5-22 and 5-23). It may expand onto the cornea in variable degrees and affect the visual axis. Usually, a pterygium develops nasally, but can occur temporally or in both areas. The causative factors are the same as for a pinguecula, namely, sun, wind, and dust exposure. In fact, a pterygium may arise from a pinguecula. When a pinguecula expands across the corneal limbus, it is called a pterygium.

A pterygium can be medically managed with lubrication, vasoconstrictors, and intermittent short courses of topical corticosteroids or NSAIDs if it becomes inflamed. Minimizing exposure to environmental factors, such as the use of ultraviolet-protective eyewear, can help reduce the growth and inflammation of a pterygium. If the lesion becomes problematic, especially if it impairs the visual axis or induces irregular astigmatism, causes recurrent irritation and redness, or impairs contact lens use, surgical excision should be considered.

Multiple different surgical procedures have been performed to try to reduce the recurrence rate of a pterygium.[12] Studies show a range in recurrence from less than 5% to as high as 90%, based on different surgical techniques and different patient populations. Currently, the safest and most effective procedure is excision of the pterygium with a free conjunctival autograft; this procedure has a recurrence rate of only

5% to 10%. Mitomycin C (MMC), in conjunction with pterygium excision, has a similar recurrence rate, but scleromalacia can occur. Beta-radiation has a slightly higher recurrence rate and more complications. Amniotic membrane grafting to bare sclera is safe, yet seems to have a slightly higher recurrence rate than does the free conjunctival autograft. The least effective procedure, excising the pterygium and leaving the sclera bare, carries a recurrence rate of more than 50%.

5-4

CONCLUSION

The management for corneal and conjunctival degeneration, particularly surgical, has been significantly improved. Excimer laser phototherapeutic keratectomy for band keratopathy, Salzmann nodular degeneration, and other anterior corneal degenerative opacities represents a new and effective treatment. Improved modalities of surgical treatment for pterygium include conjunctival graft and amniotic membrane transplantation.

REFERENCES

1. Goodfriend AN, Ching SS: Corneal and conjunctival degenerations. In: Krachmer JH, Mannis MJ, Holland EJ, eds: *Cornea: Diagnosis and Treatment.* New York: CV Mosby Co; 1997: 1119–1137.

2. Rapuano CJ, Luchs JI, Kim T, eds: *Anterior Segment: The Requisites in Ophthalmology.* St Louis: CV Mosby Co; 2000:62–102.

3. Krachmer JH, Dubord PJ, Rodrigues MM, et al: Corneal posterior crocodile shagreen and polymorphic amyloid degeneration. *Arch Ophthalmol* 1983;101:54–59.

4. O'Brart DP, Gartry DS, Lohmann CP, et al: Treatment of band keratopathy by excimer laser phototherapeutic keratectomy: surgical techniques and long term follow up. *Br J Ophthalmol* 1993;77:702–708.

5. Wood TO: Salzmann's nodular degeneration. *Cornea* 1990;9:17–22.

6. Pouliquen Y, D'Hermies F, Puech M, et al: Acute corneal edema in pellucid marginal degeneration or acute marginal keratoconus. *Cornea* 1987;6:169–174.

7. Rodrigues MM, Newsome DA, Krachmer JH, et al: Pellucid marginal corneal degeneration: a clinicopathologic study of two cases. *Exp Eye Res* 1981;33:277–288.

8. Dubroff S: Pellucid marginal corneal degeneration: report on corrective surgery. *J Cataract Refract Surg* 1989;15:89–93.

9. Barraquer-Somers E, Chan CC, Green WR: Corneal epithelial iron deposition. *Ophthalmology* 1983;90:729–734.

10. Koenig SB, McDonald MB, Yamaguchi T, et al: Corneal iron lines after refractive keratoplasty. *Arch Ophthalmol* 1983;101:1862–1865.

11. Mannis MJ: Iron deposition in the corneal graft: another corneal iron line. *Arch Ophthalmol* 1983;101:1858–1861.

12. Croasdale CR, Barney NP: Conjunctival surgery. In: Albert DM, ed: *Ophthalmic Surgery: Principles and Techniques.* Malden, MA: Blackwell Science; 1999;1:86–99.

CHAPTER 6

Excimer Laser Surgery for Corneal Dystrophies

Uyen L. Tran, MD
Ming X. Wang, MD, PhD

The treatment of anterior stromal corneal dystrophies and opacities has been greatly advanced with the introduction of excimer laser phototherapeutic keratectomy (PTK). The US Food and Drug Administration (FDA) granted the labeling of the excimer laser treatment for the cornea in the mid-to-late 1990s. The 193-nm ultraviolet light emitted by the argon fluoride (ArF) excimer laser ablates corneal tissue with submicron accuracy and with minimal damage to adjacent tissue.[1,2] By removing precise amounts of corneal tissue containing dystrophic opacities, PTK leaves an optically smooth surface, allowing basement membrane re-formation with minimal scarring.

Optimal results for PTK are obtained when the disease is confined to the anterior 100 µm of the central corneal stroma.[3] The successful removal of superficial opacities from the visual axis, with the attainment of a smooth corneal surface, can result in visual improvement. In addition, the lessening of such symptoms as glare and ocular discomfort can, in many cases, obviate the need for penetrating keratoplasty, which traditionally has been necessary in many patients who suffer from anterior stromal corneal dystrophies. When the depth of excimer laser ablation is greater than the thickness of the epithelium (about 50 µm), Bowman's layer is violated. The organization of newly formed lamellae typically takes several months and results in some anterior stromal reticular haze, which generally subsides over time.

PTK produces the most significant clinical benefit with the least amount of unpredictable iatrogenic untoward effects. When the lesion is paracentrally located, particularly if the PTK treatment area overlaps the central corneal area and involves the visual axis, the selection of location and spot size for treatment may be challenging, as laser ablative tissue removal may result in an unpredictable amount of refractive (mostly myopic) change or cause surgically induced regular or irregular astigmatism.

The many advantages of excimer laser PTK in the treatment of anterior stromal corneal dystrophy versus traditional non-laser techniques include the following:

1. At the ultrastructural level, there exists a very clear boundary between treated and untreated tissue. It has been demonstrated that adjacent areas suffer minimal distortion with no apparent thermal damage.[4]

2. Wound healing, with re-epithelialization, is rapid and is usually complete shortly after the procedure.[4]

3. The depth and diameter of treatment can be carefully controlled, enabling precise and selective removal of corneal epithelium, Bowman's layer, and anterior stromal tissue.

4. Successful removal of the anterior corneal stromal dystrophies and opacities allows patients to postpone or avoid the more invasive lamellar or penetrating keratoplasty, which carries with it the risk of rejection, graft failure, endophthalmitis, retinal detachment, or expulsive choroidal hemorrhage.

6-1

PATIENT SELECTION

Phototherapeutic keratectomy for corneal dystrophy works best when the dystrophic opacity is confined to the anterior corneal stroma.[3] PTK is also ideal if there is no significant corneal thinning. Corneal dystrophies that are amenable to treatment with PTK include epithelial and anterior stromal dystrophies, such as map-dot-fingerprint, Meesmann, Reis-Bücklers, lattice, granular, Avellino, and Schnyder, among others. PTK can also treat nondystrophic conditions, such as corneal scars resulting from infection, surgery, and trauma, or degenerative diseases, such as Salzmann nodules, keratoconus, fibroblastic nodules, and band keratopathy. Irregular corneal surfaces from pterygium surgery or spheroidal keratopathy can also be smoothed with excimer laser application.[5,6]

Contraindications to PTK for corneal dystrophies can be divided into two categories:

1. Conditions that prevent or delay wound healing

2. Conditions in which the dystrophic disease is too deep or the cornea too thin

Severe keratoconjunctivitis sicca, blepharitis, lagophthalmos, and collagen vascular diseases can potentially interfere with wound healing and re-epithelialization after laser treatment. This interference with healing can then lead to such complications as microbial keratitis, ulceration, and scarring. In eyes with thin central corneas (less than 400 μm), further tissue removal can result in a cornea that is too thin overall, leading to irregular astigmatism, postoperative haze, a large hyperopic shift, and even keratoectasia. The same is true for the treatment of deep corneal disease requiring excessive tissue removal in a cornea with no significant thinning preoperatively.

6-2

PREOPERATIVE ASSESSMENT

All patients with anterior corneal dystrophies or opacities who are considering PTK should undergo a complete ophthalmic examination, as well as a thorough review of medical history and medications. Measurements of uncorrected and best-corrected visual acuities and pupil size under mesopic conditions, as well as slit-lamp and dilated pupil examinations, are key aspects of the assessment. Examination at the slit lamp and estimation of the depth of the opacity remain the mainstay of technique in determining the level of disease. Whenever possible, preoperative corneal thickness should be measured. Slit-lamp photographs are useful in documenting the preoperative appearance of the dystrophic lesion for comparison at a later stage.

6-3

SURGICAL TECHNIQUE

The main goal of PTK is to remove the least amount of tissue necessary to achieve a clear central visual axis and smooth ocular surface. The gold standard in PTK is undertreatment. The first step in performing PTK is the removal of corneal epithelium. This can be done either with the laser or manually with a blade after 20% alcohol treatment. Kanitkar et al have shown that manual epithelium removal is less painful than laser removal.[7] The decision is also based on the condition of Bowman's layer. If Bowman's layer is smooth relative to the epithelium, then epithelial removal can be done manually. Any irregularities of Bowman's layer in the setting of a relatively smooth epithelial surface call for removal with the excimer laser, with the epithelium serving as a natural masking agent for smooth ablation.

A large-diameter treatment zone (typically, 6 to 6.5 mm) is centered over the entrance pupil and the epithelium, and as much of the confluent dystrophic opacity is removed as possible. Treatment is halted if an irregular or elevated lesion is encountered, and masking gel fluid (for example, nitrocellulose 1%) is then applied. Deeper lesions should not be ablated, as deep laser treatment itself can cause scar formation or a large hyperopic shift. Patients should be repeatedly examined at the slit lamp during the treatment session to determine if more treatment is necessary. In general, the main guideline for PTK is to undertreat and then to repeat treatment if needed.

For irregular dystrophic opacities, masking gel fluids are extremely important for achieving a smooth surface once the stromal layer is reached. Their role is to fill in depressions while exposing elevations of an irregular surface. The most important principle is to use the least amount of fluid required to cover the valleys, as too much fluid can alter ablation depth. Many agents of varying viscosities are available.[8] Hydroxy-propylmethylcellulose 0.1% with dextran is of low viscosity and may leave the valleys, as well as the peaks, partly exposed. Car-boxylmethylcellulose 0.5% is of medium viscosity and effectively covers the valleys while exposing the peaks. Healon and 1% to 2% methylcellulose are of high viscosity and may cover the peaks as well as the valleys. Multiple agents or a combination can be selectively used based on the surface irregularities encountered.

PTK has been shown to be a safe and effective alternative for the treatment of anterior corneal dystrophies, such as anterior basement membrane, Meesmann, Reis-Bücklers, lattice, granular, and Avellino.[5,9–12] For corneal dystrophies or opacities located deep in the corneal stroma, such as macular corneal dystrophy, PTK has limited efficacy. The recurrence rate after PTK with the excimer laser is similar to that after manual scraping or corneal transplantation. Recurrences after PTK can be re-treated with a high degree of success. The same PTK technique can be applied to recurrences of anterior stromal corneal dystrophy in penetrating keratoplasty patients, although the chance of PTK-induced corneal scarring is somewhat higher in the graft possibly because of central corneal denervation after penetrating keratoplasty and delayed epithelial healing in many cases.

PTK can also be used to treat complications after excimer laser photorefractive keratectomy (PRK). Post-PRK complications include irregular astigmatism, decentered ablation, and anterior stromal corneal scarring.[13–16] Irregular astigmatism after PRK can be ameliorated with PTK by using a masking agent or by customizing treatment of the steep areas of the cornea as identified by topography.[17]

6-4

POSTOPERATIVE CARE

In the immediate post-PTK period, a bandage contact lens is placed, along with instillation of a broad-spectrum antibiotic and nonsteroidal drops. Patients are instructed to use these drops 4 times a day, along with the copious use of nonpreserved artificial tears, until the epithelial defect has healed. Patients are examined every 24 to 72 hours until the cornea has completely re-epithelialized. Followup is usually at 1 month, 3 months, 6 months, and 1 year, with annual examinations thereafter. The role of postoperative topical corticosteroids in reducing post-PTK scarring has not been established.

6-5

SIDE EFFECTS AND COMPLICATIONS

6-5-1 Pain

In the first 24 to 48 hours, pain may be severe. As mentioned earlier, at least one study demonstrated that manual epithelium removal is less painful than laser removal.[7] The discomfort is lessened with the use of bandage contact lenses and nonsteroidal drops. Narcotic pain medications, nonsteroid oral medications, or tranquilizers can also be prescribed as needed. The pain usually dissipates quickly as the epithelium heals, which generally occurs in 1 week. In patients with concurrent band keratopathy,

Salzmann nodular degeneration, or severe dry eye, re-epithelialization may take 3 to 4 weeks.[18] Adjunctive therapy, such as temporary lateral tarsorrhaphy and punctal occlusion (silicone plugs or cautery), may assist with healing.

6-5-2 Refractive Shifts

The most common refractive change after PTK is the induced hyperopia from laser tissue removal of the central cornea. It has been hypothesized that the excimer laser beam is directed perpendicular to the central cornea, but treats the peripheral cornea at an angle that ablates less tissue.[14-16] In addition, epithelial and stromal hyperplasia, along with a flatter tear meniscus in the periphery, may result in greater peripheral tissue filling and thus relative central corneal flattening. The periphery may also be shielded by ablation evaporative products.

Strategies to decrease the induced hyperopia have met with some success. Sher et al performed PTK with a rotating circular approach under the laser beam of varying aperture size.[10] Hyperopic ablations can also be performed following PTK to correct the hyperopic shift. Stark et al[1] and Chamon et al[18] have treated the ablation margins with a modified taper technique, using an annulus with a 2.0-mm diameter and limiting depth to 20 μm. Utilizing appropriate masking agents and limiting treatment depth can prevent large visually significant hyperopic changes.

With respect to the amount of hyperopic shift after a central PTK treatment zone 6 mm in diameter, Rathod et al conducted a study of 17 consecutive eyes; the mean hyperopic shift without masking agent was 1.78 D (range: 0.125 to 5 D).[19] The average stromal ablation depth per diopter change was about 42 μm/D. Conversely, central 6-mm PTK created a shift of 0.024 D per 1-μm depth of corneal tissue removal. From the study, the authors derived the following mathematical relationship between post-PTK hyperopic shift (D, in diopters) and stromal ablation depth (SAD, in microns):

$$D = SAD/42$$

Myopia can also be induced with PTK in the treatment of a paracentral opacity. In these cases, the peripheral or paracentral cornea undergoes a deeper ablation than does the central cornea. The myopic shift has been noted in 3% to 16% of patients undergoing PTK.[10,20]

Irregular astigmatism is another unwanted refractive change that can occur after PTK. It can be the result of a decentered ablation or of an irregular postoperative corneal contour, particularly in some patients with anterior dystrophic opacities that are elevated preoperatively. Masking agents can help to achieve a smooth corneal surface after treatment. Centration of the laser and proper patient fixation are critical to a successful outcome. The preoperative use of miotics is discouraged, as miotics can cause decentered displacement of the pupil, resulting in a decentered ablation if the laser was aimed at the pupil.

6-5-3 Induced Haze and Scarring

Scarring that significantly impairs vision after a properly performed PTK is rare. Immediately after laser ablation, a reticular haze can be noted; the haze usually subsides in 3 to 6 months. The use of topical corticosteroids can minimize the duration and severity of postoperative haze. Significant scarring is usually the result of an ablation that extends too deep. In general, PTK treatment should not extend beyond 100 μm. The minimum residual total corneal thickness should be *at least* 400 μm. A thinner total corneal thickness can lead to long-term complications, such as significant scarring, instability, and corneal ectasia. Treating post-PRK scarring in conjunction with mitomycin C is undergoing active investigation. Patients with visually significant corneal scarring and haze after PTK may benefit from lamellar or penetrating keratoplasty.

6-5-4 Infectious Keratitis

Bacterial infectious keratitis can occur following PTK. Predisposing factors include ocular surface disease, the prolonged presence of an epithelial defect, the placement of a contact lens on what may be an already immunocompromised ocular surface, and the use of postoperative corticosteroids. Prophylaxis against infections is achieved with the use of postoperative topical antibiotics until the epithelial defect is healed, with prompt removal of the bandage contact lens. Most ophthalmologists believe that the ability of the bandage contact lens to promote healing and ameliorate pain outweighs the risk of infection. Corneal infiltrates are managed aggressively in a similar protocol to that used for patients who have

not had laser treatment. When PTK is used to treat a scar from herpes simplex keratitis, reactivation of the latent virus may occur[12,21,22] so the use of antivirals preoperatively and postoperatively is prudent.[20]

6-5-5 Corneal Graft Rejection

Indications for PTK in patients who have undergone penetrating keratoplasty include recurrence of the corneal dystrophy on the graft. Treatment is performed with caution, however, as graft rejection has been reported to occur postoperatively.[23,24] A reversal of the rejection can be accomplished by aggressive topical or systemic immunosuppression. The use of corticosteroids is important, but should be delayed until complete corneal re-epithelialization of the graft has occurred.

6-6

CLINICAL OUTCOMES

PTK treatment for anterior stromal corneal dystrophy has been shown to be both safe and effective. Figures 6-1 and 6-2 show two examples of successful PTK treatment for corneal dystrophies. Two large multicenter trials were performed to evaluate the efficacy and safety of PTK for corneal dystrophies and anterior stromal opacities due to other causes.[25,26] The VISX study consisted of 269 eyes that underwent primary PTK in 17 centers. Best spectacle-corrected visual acuity (BSCVA) improved by at least 2 lines in 53% of eyes and by at least 3 lines in 41% at 1 year. Conversely, 8% lost 2 or more lines, while 6.8% lost 3 or more lines at the 1-year mark. The average refractive shift was 2.3 diopters at 1 year.

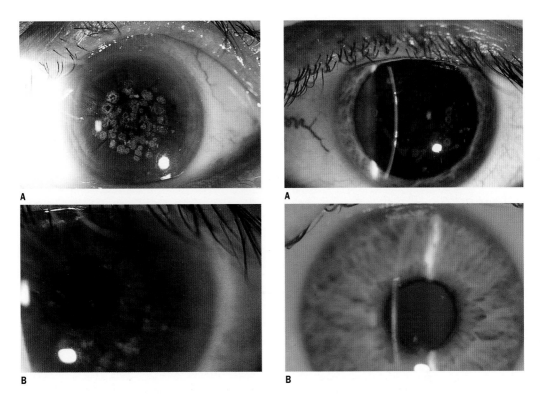

Figure 6-1 *PTK treatment of granular corneal dystrophy. (A) Preoperative appearance. Best-corrected vision was 20/50 in this eye, with complaint of haze and glare. (B) Postoperative appearance (2 years after PTK). Most of central dystrophic opacity has been removed. Best-corrected vision improved to 20/25.*

Figure 6-2 *PTK treatment of anterior stromal corneal dystrophy. (A) Preoperative appearance. Slit beam shows anterior stromal granular opacity. (B) Postoperative appearance (6 months after PTK).*

The Summit Technology Excimer Laser Study included a total of 398 eyes. The proportion of patients who had at least 20/40 BSCVA increased by 22% at 1 year. Further, the percentage of patients who had 20/100 or worse BSCVA decreased by 10%. About 73% of patients achieved success, as defined by an increase in 2 or more lines of BSCVA or a significant decrease in subjective complaints from patients who underwent PTK for improved comfort. Of the patients who responded to a questionnaire, 85% said they would undergo PTK again.

CONCLUSION

The 193-nm argon fluoride (ArF) excimer laser has been shown to be safe and effective in treating epithelial and anterior stromal corneal dystrophies and opacities. The use of PTK may delay or avoid altogether the risk and expense of more invasive procedures, such as corneal transplantation. To maintain safety, however, the limitations of the procedure must be emphasized. The cardinal rule of PTK is to treat the least amount of tissue necessary to clear the visual axis. Deep corneal lesions should not be treated, as deep PTK treatment itself induces scar formation and corneal thinning. The use of masking fluids is helpful to achieve a smooth corneal surface and reduce the incidence of irregular astigmatism. Corneal dystrophies may recur after PTK treatment or after penetrating keratoplasty, and additional PTK treatment can be effective. Treatment must be individualized, depending on the nature of the disease and its ablation characteristics and depth.

Central PTK can cause hyperopic shift, which needs to be taken into account particularly if patients are in the presbyopic age range. The success of PTK in the treatment of anterior corneal opacities due to corneal dystrophies and other conditions has been demonstrated in multiple large clinical trials. Treating corneal scarring with PTK in conjunction with mitomycin C is being actively investigated. PTK adds an exciting and effective treatment modality to the armamentarium of corneal surgeons in the management of anterior corneal dystrophies and opacities.

REFERENCES

1. Stark WJ, Chamon W, Kamp MT, et al: Clinical follow-up of 193-nm ArF excimer laser photokeratectomy. *Ophthalmology* 1992;99:805–812.

2. Gaster RN, Binder PS, Coalwell K, et al: Corneal surface ablation by 193 nm excimer laser and wound healing in rabbits. *Invest Ophthalmol Vis Sci* 1989;30:90–98.

3. Marshall J, Trokel S, Rothery S, et al: Photoablative reprofiling of the cornea using an excimer laser: photorefractive keratectomy. *Lasers Ophthalmol* 1986;1:23–44.

4. Marshall J, Trokel S, Rothery S, et al: A comparative study of corneal incisions induced by diamond and steel knives and two ultraviolet radiations from an excimer laser. *Br J Ophthalmol* 1986;70:482–501.

5. Ohman L, Fagerholm P, Tengroth B: Treatment of recurrent corneal erosions with the excimer laser. *Acta Ophthalmol* 1994;72:461–463.

6. Hersh PR, Spinak A, Garrana R, et al: Phototherapeutic keratectomy: strategies and results in 12 eyes. *Refract Corneal Surg* 1993;9(suppl): S90–S94.

7. Kanitkar KD, Camp J, Humble H, et al: Pain after epithelial removal by ethanol-assisted mechanical versus transepithelial excimer laser debridement. *J Refract Surg* 2000;16:519–522.

8. Kornmehl EW, Steinert RF, Puliafito CA: A comparative study of masking fluids for excimer laser phototherapeutic keratectomy. *Arch Ophthalmol* 1991;109:860–863.

9. Orndahl M, Fagerholm P, Fitzsimmons T, et al: Treatment of corneal dystrophies with excimer laser. *Acta Ophthalmol* 1994;72:235–240.

10. Sher NA, Bowers RA, Zabel RW, et al: Clinical use of 193-nm excimer laser in the treatment of corneal scars. *Arch Ophthalmol* 1991;109:491–498.

11. Forster W, Grewe S, Atzler U, et al: Phototherapeutic keratectomy in corneal diseases. *Refract Corneal Surg* 1993;9(suppl):S85–S89.

12. Fagerholm P, Fitzsimmons TD, Orndahl M, et al: Phototherapeutic keratectomy: long-term results in 166 eyes. *Refract Corneal Surg* 1993; 9(suppl 2):76–81.

13. Rachid MD, Yoo SH, Azar DT: Phototherapeutic keratectomy for decentration and central islands after photorefractive keratectomy. *Ophthalmology* 2001;108:545–552.

14. Azar DT, Yeh PC: Corneal topographic evaluation in decentration in photorefractive keratectomy: treatment displacement vs intraoperative drift. *Am J Ophthalmol* 1997;124:312–320.

15. Azar DT, Stark WJ, Steinert RF: Surgical management of PRK complications. In: Azar DT, Steinert RF, Stark WJ: *Excimer Laser Phototherapeutic Keratectomy.* Baltimore, MD: Williams & Wilkins; 1997:169–172.

16. Azar DT, Talamo JH, Helena MC, et al: PTK: indications, surgical techniques, postoperative care, and complications management. In: Talamo JH, Kreuger RR, eds: *The Excimer Manual: A Clinician's Guide to Excimer Laser Surgery.* Boston: Little, Brown; 1997:173–198.

17. Gibralter R, Trokel SL: Correction of irregular astigmatism with the excimer laser. *Ophthalmology* 1994;101:1310–1314.

18. Chamon W, Azar DT, Stark WJ, et al: Phototherapeutic keratectomy. *Ophthalmol Clin North Am* 1993;6:399–413.

19. Rathod R, Shen DJ, Wang MX: Relationship between stromal ablation depth and hyperopic shift after 6 mm phototherapeutic keratectomy using VISX Star excimer laser. *Invest Ophthalmol Vis Sci* 2002;43:B134.

20. Campos M, Nielson S, Szerenyi K, et al: Clinical follow-up of phototherapeutic keratectomy for treatment of corneal opacities. *Am J Ophthalmol* 1993;115:433–440.

21. Vrabec MP, Anderson JA, Rock ME, et al: Electron microscopic findings in a cornea with recurrence of herpes simplex keratitis after excimer laser phototherapeutic keratectomy. *CLAO J* 1994;20:41–44.

22. Pepose JS, Laycock KA, Miller JK, et al: Reactivation of latent herpes simplex virus by excimer laser photokeratectomy. *Am J Ophthalmol* 1992;114:45–50.

23. Hersh PS, Jordan AJ, Mayers M: Corneal graft rejection episode after excimer laser phototherapeutic keratectomy. *Arch Ophthalmol* 1993; 11:735–736.

24. Epstein RJ, Robin JB: Corneal graft rejection episode after excimer laser phototherapeutic keratectomy. *Arch Ophthalmol* 1994;112:157.

25. Ashraf F, Azar D, Odrich M: Clinical results of PTK using the VISX excimer laser. In: Azar DT, Steinert RF, Stark WJ: *Excimer Laser Phototherapeutic Keratectomy.* Baltimore, MD: Williams & Wilkins; 1997:201–205.

26. Steinert RF: Clinical results with the Summit Technology excimer laser. In: Azar DT, Steinert RF, Stark WJ: *Excimer Laser Phototherapeutic Keratectomy.* Baltimore, MD: Williams & Wilkins; 1997:155–156.

OPHTHALMOLOGY MONOGRAPH 16
Corneal Dystrophies and Degenerations: A Molecular Genetics Approach

CME Accreditation
The American Academy of Ophthalmology is accredited by the Accreditation Council for Continuing Medical Education to provide continuing medical education for physicians.

The American Academy of Ophthalmology designates this educational activity for a maximum of 20 hours in category 1 credit toward the AMA Physician's Recognition Award. Each physician should claim only those hours of credit that he/she has actually spent in the activity.

CME Credit Report Forms
If you wish to claim CME credit for your study of this monograph, you must send this page and the following three pages (by mail or fax) to the Academy office. Please make sure to:

1. Fill in and sign the statement below.
2. Write your answers to the questions on the back of this page.
3. Complete the self-study examination and mark your answers on the answer sheet.
4. Complete the product evaluation.

Important These completed forms must be received at the Academy within 3 years of purchase.

I hereby certify that I have spent _____ (up to 20) hours of study on this monograph and that I have completed the self-study examination. (The Academy, upon request, will send you a verification of your Academy credits earned within the last 3 years.)

Signature   Date

PLEASE PRINT

Last Name   First Name   MI

Mailing Address

City

State   ZIP Code

Telephone   ID Number*

Please return the completed forms to:

> **American Academy of Ophthalmology**
> **P.O. Box 7424**
> **San Francisco, CA 94120-7424**
> **ATTN: Clinical Education Division**

*Your ID Number is located following your name on most Academy mailing labels, in your member directory, and on your monthly statement of account.

OPHTHALMOLOGY MONOGRAPH 16
Corneal Dystrophies and Degenerations: A Molecular Genetics Approach

1. Please list several ways in which your study of this monograph will affect your practice.

_____

_____

_____

_____

_____

_____

_____

2. How can we improve this monograph to better meet your continuing medical education needs?

_____

_____

_____

_____

_____

_____

_____

3. *Optional* Please list any topics you would like to see covered in other Academy clinical education products.

_____

_____

_____

_____

_____

_____

_____

OPHTHALMOLOGY MONOGRAPH 16
Corneal Dystrophies and Degenerations: A Molecular Genetics Approach

Circle the letter of the response option that you regard as the "best" answer to the question.

Question	Answer			
1	a	b	c	d
2	a	b	c	d
3	a	b	c	d
4	a	b	c	d
5	a	b	c	d
6	a	b	c	d
7	a	b	c	d
8	a	b	c	d
9	a	b	c	d
10	a	b	c	d
11	a	b	c	d
12	a	b	c	d
13	a	b	c	d
14	a	b	c	d
15	a	b	c	d
16	a	b	c	d

Please complete the product evaluation on the back of this page.

PLEASE CUT ALONG DASHED LINE

OPHTHALMOLOGY MONOGRAPH 16
Corneal Dystrophies and Degenerations: A Molecular Genetics Approach

Please indicate your response to the statements listed below by placing the appropriate number to the left of each statement.

1 = Agree strongly

2 = Agree

3 = No opinion

4 = Disagree

5 = Disagree strongly

_____ This monograph meets its stated objectives.

_____ This monograph helped me keep current on this topic.

_____ I will apply knowledge gained from this monograph to my practice.

_____ This monograph covers topics in sufficient depth and detail.

_____ This monograph's illustrations are of sufficient number and quality.

_____ The references included in the monograph provide an appropriate amount of additional reading.

_____ The self-study examination at the end of the monograph is useful.

SELF-STUDY EXAMINATION

The self-study examination provided for each book in the Ophthalmology Monographs series is intended for use after completion of the monograph. The examination for *Corneal Dystrophies and Degenerations: A Molecular Genetics Approach* consists of 16 multiple-choice questions followed by the answers to the questions and a discussion for each answer. The Academy recommends that you not consult the answers until you have completed the entire examination.

Questions

The questions are constructed so that there is one "best" answer. Despite the attempt to avoid ambiguous selections, disagreement may occur about which selection constitutes the optimal answer. After reading a question, record your initial impression on the answer sheet.

Answers and Discussions

The "best" answer to each question is provided after the examination. The discussion that accompanies the answer is intended to help you confirm that the reasoning you used in determining the most appropriate answer was correct. If you missed a question, the discussion may help you decide whether your "error" was due to poor wording of the question or to your misinterpretation. If, instead, you missed the question because of miscalculation or failure to recall relevant information, the discussion may help fix the principle in your memory.

QUESTIONS

Chapter 1

1. The gene that has been identified on human chromosome 5q31 and that is involved in anterior stromal corneal dystrophies is named
   a. *TGFBI*
   b. *BIGH3*
   c. keratoepithelin
   d. all of the above

2. The most common type of DNA mutation found in 5q31-linked anterior corneal stromal dystrophies is
   a. deletion
   b. point mutation
   c. duplication
   d. inversion

Chapter 2

3. Which of the following corneal dystrophies is caused by defects in keratin genes?
   a. Reis-Bücklers corneal dystrophy
   b. honeycomb corneal dystrophy of Thiel-Behnke
   c. Meesmann epithelial corneal dystrophy
   d. map-dot-fingerprint dystrophy

4. Which of the following corneal dystrophies is(are) inherited in an autosomal dominant fashion?
   a. Meesmann epithelial corneal dystrophy
   b. Lisch corneal dystrophy
   c. Reis-Bücklers corneal dystrophy
   d. a and c

Chapter 3

5. Subtypes of lattice corneal dystrophies involve genetic loci on the following human chromosomes:
   a. 5 and 9
   b. 5 and 1
   c. 9 and 1
   d. 12 and 17

6. Which of the following diseases has an autosomal recessive inheritance pattern?

   a. lattice type I

   b. macular corneal dystrophy

   c. granular corneal dystrophy

   d. Avellino corneal dystrophy

Chapter 4

7. A 65-year-old retired Caucasian female presents to your office with a chief complaint of blurry vision upon awakening. She has a history of mild myopia, for which she wears corrective lenses. Her past ocular history is otherwise unremarkable. Her best-corrected spectacle visual acuity is 20/20 in both eyes. On ophthalmic examination, there is evidence for bilateral central corneal guttae without stromal edema, as well as early nuclear sclerotic cataracts. The rest of the ophthalmic examination is unremarkable. All of the following are appropriate management options *except*

   a. topical hyperosmotic agents (5% sodium chloride)

   b. corneal dehydration with a blow-dryer held at arm's length

   c. penetrating keratoplasty without cataract removal

   d. a search for other contributing factors

8. Which of the following characterizes congenital hereditary endothelial dystrophy (CHED)?

   a. markedly decreased corneal thickness

   b. functionally and morphologically abnormal corneal endothelial cells

   c. central corneal guttae

   d. multilayered endothelium

9. Which of the following characterizes posterior polymorphous dystrophy (PPMD)?

   a. autosomal recessive inheritance pattern

   b. progressive corneal clouding requiring corneal transplantation

   c. frequently associated with secondary glaucoma

   d. normal corneal thickness

10. Visual prognosis in the iridocorneal endothelial (ICE) syndrome is best determined by

   a. absence of corneal edema

   b. absence of iris lesions

   c. adequate glaucoma control

   d. early surgical intervention

Chapter 5

11. All of the following are characteristics of pellucid marginal degeneration *except*

a. absence of Bowman's layer

b. against-the-rule astigmatism

c. hydrops

d. Vogt's striae

12. Corneal thinning occurs in all of the following conditions *except*

a. Terrien marginal degeneration

b. band keratopathy

c. furrow degeneration

d. pellucid marginal degeneration

13. Astigmatism can be induced by all of the following conditions *except*

a. polymorphic amyloid deposition

b. pellucid marginal degeneration

c. pterygium

d. Terrien marginal degeneration

14. The main treatment for band keratopathy is

a. phototherapeutic keratectomy (PTK)

b. superficial keratectomy

c. Na-EDTA

d. penetrating keratoplasty

Chapter 6

15. Corneal dystrophies that can be treated with phototherapeutic keratectomy (PTK) include all of the following *except*

a. map-dot-fingerprint dystrophy

b. Meesmann epithelial corneal dystrophy

c. macular corneal dystrophy

d. Reis-Bücklers corneal dystrophy

16. In phototherapeutic keratectomy (PTK), masking gel agents are used

a. to fill in depressions while exposing elevations for irregular opacities

b. as wetting agents for the corneal epithelium

c. to remove debris from the ocular surface

d. as a comfort measure postoperatively

ANSWERS AND DISCUSSIONS

Chapter 1

1. **Answer—d.** All three names have been used to designate this gene. *TGFBI* = transforming growth factor beta-induced. *BIGH3* = beta-induced gene human cell clone number 3.

2. **Answer—b.** The majority of the DNA mutations found in *TGFBI* are DNA point mutations. These mutations result in a substitution of one amino acid by another, causing changes in three-dimensional structure of the protein and resulting in dystrophic precipitations.

Chapter 2

3. **Answer—c.** Meesmann epithelial corneal dystrophy is caused by mutations in either of the genes encoding keratins K3 or K12. Reis-Bücklers corneal dystrophy and honeycomb dystrophy of Thiel-Behnke are caused by specific mutations in the *TGFBI* gene. Map-dot-fingerprint dystrophy (MDFD or epithelial basement membrane dystrophy) is of unknown causation.

4. **Answer—d.** Meesmann epithelial corneal dystrophy (MECD) and Reis-Bücklers corneal dystrophy (RBCD) are inherited in an autosomal dominant fashion. The molecular basis of MECD is known to be mutations in either keratin 3 or keratin 12, and RBCD is known to be due to mutations in the *TGFBI* gene. Lisch corneal dystrophy is X-linked, and while the genetic basis is as yet unknown, it has been mapped to xp22.3.

Chapter 3

5. **Answer—a.** Human chromosome 5q31 contains the *TGFBI* gene, which is implicated in lattice types I and IIIA, granular, and Avellino corneal dystrophies; 9q34 contains the gelsolin gene, which is implicated in lattice type II corneal dystrophy; 1p31 contains the *M1S1* gene, which is implicated in gelatinous drop-like corneal dystrophy; 12q13 and 17q12 contain keratin genes 3 and 12, respectively, which are implicated in Meesmann epithelial corneal dystrophy.

6. **Answer—b.** Macular corneal dystrophy is the only disease listed that has an autosomal recessive inheritance pattern.

Chapter 4

7. Answer—c. Although penetrating kerato-plasty is the definitive treatment of choice for Fuchs endothelial dystrophy, it should be performed only in more advanced cases or when there is impairment of vision sufficient to interfere with activities of daily living. Hyperosmotic agents, as well as corneal dehydration by various methods, are accepted medical treatments for early Fuchs dystrophy. Other causes for decreased vision upon awakening should be addressed and treated (for example, blepharitis), in addition to the dystrophy.

8. Answer—b. Decreased corneal thickness is not a feature of the corneal endothelial dystrophies. Corneal guttae are found in Fuchs dystrophy, not in congenital hereditary endothelial dystrophy (CHED). Multilayered endothelium is a feature of posterior polymorphous dystrophy (PPMD), not of CHED.

9. Answer—d. Posterior polymorphous dystrophy (PPMD) is inherited as an autosomal dominant trait. Slow progression or no progression is the rule, with corneal transplantation being an infrequent occurrence. Although secondary glaucoma may be associated with PPMD, it is not a common finding (15%). Peripheral anterior synechiae and secondary glaucoma denote a worse prognosis for patients with PPMD.

10. Answer—c. The key determinant in the ultimate visual prognosis of the iridocorneal endothelial (ICE) syndrome is adequate control of glaucoma, whether this requires medical or surgical management.

Chapter 5

11. Answer—d. Pellucid marginal degeneration causes thinning in the corneal stroma and an absence of Bowman's layer on histopathology. It results in against-the-rule astigmatism, and hydrops may occur. Vogt's striae is characteristic of keratoconus. The lack of Vogt's striae in pellucid marginal degeneration can be used to differentiate keratoconus from pellucid marginal degeneration.

12. **Answer—b.** In Terrien marginal degeneration, thinning occurs in the supranasal peripheral cornea and extends circumferentially or centrally. Furrow degeneration causes thinning between the corneal limbus and arcus. Pellucid marginal degeneration usually causes thinning in the inferior cornea. Band keratopathy is not usually associated with corneal thinning.

13. **Answer—a.** Polymorphic amyloid deposition does not induce astigmatism because it usually occurs diffusely in the cornea. Terrien marginal degeneration and pellucid marginal degeneration cause corneal thinning and induce astigmatism. If a pterygium extends onto the central cornea, astigmatism may be induced.

14. **Answer—c.** Na-EDTA is the most effective treatment for band keratopathy because it chelates calcium. Superficial keratectomy can be used to remove large calcium pieces. Phototherapeutic keratectomy (PTK) may be performed for recurrent band keratopathy.

Chapter 6

15. **Answer—c.** Macular corneal dystrophy is not amenable to treatment with phototherapeutic keratectomy (PTK), as the lesions can extend to Descemet's membrane and the endothelium. PTK gives the best results when the disease is confined to the anterior 100 μm of the cornea.

16. **Answer—a.** Masking gel agents are extremely important in achieving a smooth ablation for irregular opacities. The most important principle is to use the least amount of fluid necessary to cover the valleys, because too much fluid can alter ablation depth.

INDEX

NOTE: An *f* following a page number indicates a figure, and a *t* following a page number indicates a table.

END USER LICENSE AGREEMENT

IMPORTANT: READ BEFORE OPENING OR USING THE DISKETTE!

This is a software license agreement ("Agreement") between you, as the end user, and the American Academy of Ophthalmology, Inc., a Minnesota nonprofit corporation ("the Academy"). BY OPENING THE SEALED DISKETTE PACKAGE, YOU AGREE THAT YOU HAVE READ THE AGREEMENT, THAT YOU UNDERSTAND IT, THAT YOU AGREE TO ITS TERMS, AND THAT IT IS THE ONLY AGREEMENT BETWEEN YOU AND THE ACADEMY ABOUT THE CD-ROM. If you do not agree to the following terms, return the diskette package unused and unopened to the Academy, at 655 Beach Street, P.O. Box 7424, San Francisco, California 94120, for a full refund.

1. *Grant of License* The Academy grants you a nonexclusive license to use the enclosed software ("Software") on computers owned or leased by you for your own use as an individual physician or eyecare provider.

2. *Ownership* The Academy owns or licenses the CD-ROM, including any adaptations or copies, and you will not have any ownership rights in them. A copy is provided to you only to allow you to exercise your rights under this License Agreement.

3. *Copies* The CD-ROM is copyrighted. You may download the images on the CD-ROM to your own computer, but any other reproduction or use is prohibited without the written permission of the American Academy of Ophthalmology.

4. *Other Restrictions* Except as described in Section 1 of this License, you may not transfer, rent, sublicense, or otherwise distribute all or any part of the CD-ROM. The Images or copies of the Images cannot be resold, used in any materials that will be sold, or used to market any products or materials being sold.

5. *Limited Warranty* The Academy warrants that the CD-ROM is free from defects in workmanship for 90 days from the date of purchase. The Academy will replace defective CD-ROMs upon receipt of the CD-ROM and proof of payment. This warranty does not cover defects due to accident, abuse, modification, or any other cause occurring after you have opened the CD-ROM package.

6. *NO OTHER WARRANTIES* TO THE MAXIMUM EXTENT PERMITTED BY APPLICABLE LAW, THE ACADEMY AND ITS LICENSORS DISCLAIM ALL OTHER WARRANTIES, EITHER EXPRESS OR IMPLIED, INCLUDING, BUT NOT LIMITED TO, IMPLIED WARRANTIES OF MERCHANTABILITY AND FITNESS FOR A PARTICULAR PURPOSE, WITH REGARD TO THE CD-ROM. SOME STATES DO NOT ALLOW EXCLUDING OR LIMITING IMPLIED WARRANTIES, SO THIS LIMITATION MAY NOT APPLY TO YOU.

7. *LIMITATION OF LIABILITY* IN NO EVENT WILL THE ACADEMY BE LIABLE FOR ANY DIRECT, INDIRECT, INCIDENTAL, SPECIAL, CONSEQUENTIAL, OR OTHER DAMAGES ARISING OUT OF THE USE OF THE CD-ROM BY ANY PERSON, WHETHER OR NOT INFORMED OF THE POSSIBILITY OF DAMAGES IN ADVANCE. THE ACADEMY'S TOTAL LIABILITY WITH RESPECT TO ALL CAUSES OF ACTION TOGETHER WILL NOT EXCEED THE AMOUNT YOU PAID THE ACADEMY FOR THIS LICENSE. THESE LIMITATIONS APPLY TO ALL CAUSES OF ACTION, INCLUDING BREACH OF CONTRACT, BREACH OF WARRANTY, THE ACADEMY'S NEGLIGENCE, STRICT LIABILITY, MISREPRESENTATION, AND OTHER TORTS. SOME STATES DO NOT ALLOW THE EXCLUSION OR LIMITATION OF INCIDENTAL OR CONSEQUENTIAL DAMAGES, SO THE ABOVE LIMITATIONS OR EXCLUSIONS MAY NOT APPLY TO YOU.

8. *Term* This License will become effective on the date you acquire the CD-ROM and will remain in force until terminated. You may terminate this License at any time by destroying the CD-ROM and all copies. This License also will automatically terminate if you breach any of these terms or conditions. You agree to destroy the original and all copies of the CD-ROM, or to return them to the Academy, upon termination of this License.

9. *U.S. Government Restricted Rights* Use, reproduction, or disclosure by the U.S. Government is subject to restrictions as set forth in FAR′ 52.227-14 Alt III, FAR′ 52.227-19, or DFARS′ 227.7202-3, as applicable.

SYSTEM REQUIREMENTS

For PC

- Personal computer using Pentium® 166-MHz processor or faster
- Microsoft® Windows™ 95 or later
- 800 × 600 monitor, 16-bit resolution (thousands of colors)
- CD-ROM drive, 4X-speed minimum
- Mouse or compatible pointing device

For Macintosh

- Apple Macintosh® computer, 120-MHz PowerPC™ or faster
- Apple Macintosh System 8.1 or later
- 800 × 600 monitor, 16-bit resolution (thousands of colors)
- CD-ROM drive, 4X-speed minimum
- Mouse or compatible pointing device

Pentium is a registered trademark of Intel Corporation. Microsoft is a registered trademark and Windows is a trademark of Microsoft Corporation. Apple, Macintosh, and System 8 are trademarks of Apple Computer, Inc. PowerPC is a trademark of International Business Machines Corporation.